MCQs for Part 2 MRCOG

DAVID J OWEN
MRCOG
Senior Registrar
Liverpool Women's Hospital, Liverpool

and

MUHAMMAD A AKHTAR
MRCOG
Senior Registrar
Research Fellow in Reproductive Medicine
University of Warwick
University Hospitals of Coventry and Warwickshire

Forewords by
SANJEEV D SHARMA
MD, FRCOG
Consultant Obstetrician and Gynaecologist
Director of Medical Education
Southport and Ormskirk Hospital NHS Trust

and

YASMIN SAJJAD
MBBS, MRCOG, MD
Consultant Gynaecologist and Andrologist
Subspecialist in Reproductive Medicine and Surgery
St Mary's Hospital, Central Manchester Foundation Trust

Radcliffe Publishing
London • New York

Radcliffe Publishing Ltd
33–41 Dallington Street
London
EC1V 0BB
United Kingdom

www.radcliffepublishing.com

British Library Cataloguing in Publication Data

A catalogue record for this book is available from the British Library.

ISBN-13: 978 184619 591 4

The paper used for the text pages of this book
is FSC® certified. FSC (The Forest Stewardship
Council®) is an international network to promote
responsible management of the world's forests.

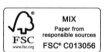

Typeset by Beautiful Words, Auckland, New Zealand
Printed and bound by TJI Digital, Padstow, Cornwall, UK

Contents

Foreword

The MRCOG Part 2 written examination includes multiple-choice questions (MCQs), extended matching questions (EMQs) and short essay questions (SAQs). MCQs constitute 30% of the written examination and are included to test a candidate's breadth of knowledge. The successful candidate not only has the knowledge but also understands the technique required to answer the MCQs.

This book provides trainees in obstetrics and gynaecology with an overview of the whole syllabus for the Part 2 examination. The questions have been divided according to modules as described in the curriculum. The authors have written completely new questions, included helpful hints in the explanations and have been careful to achieve both general and specific validity by detailed blueprinting of the curriculum. The questions have been extensively sourced from the RCOG's suggested reading material.

The book will provide excellent revision material for trainees and will enable them to consolidate their knowledge and teach them the techniques required to successfully answer the questions.

I would recommend this book to all trainees preparing for the Part 2 examination.

Sanjeev D Sharma MD, FRCOG
Consultant Obstetrician and Gynaecologist
Director of Medical Education
Southport and Ormskirk Hospital NHS Trust
June 2012

Foreword

The MRCOG Part 2 examination is one of the most difficult postgraduate exams, with a success rate of less than 30%. Preparing for this examination remains a multifaceted task, particularly as learning and revision often needs to fit around the trainee's shift work, on call status and other busy clinical commitments.

From March 2011, the format of the Part 2 MRCOG written examination has changed. The number of MCQs and EMQs has increased.

MCQs are designed to test a candidate's theoretical and practical knowledge of obstetrics and gynaecology. Therefore, it is crucial that a candidate acquires experience and practice in answering them beforehand.

This book concentrates on the core areas of the syllabus. All the answers are evidence based, in line with the guidelines published by the RCOG, the National Institute for Health and Clinical Excellence (NICE) and the most up-to-date consensus.

With a wide and varied selection of practice MCQs, this book will prepare candidates to effectively answer any type of MCQs. The book will be an invaluable addition to the bookshelves of all those candidates who are planning to take the MRCOG Part 2. I would highly recommend it to any trainee intending to sit the final part of the MRCOG exam.

Yasmin Sajjad MBBS, MRCOG, MD
Consultant Gynaecologist and Andrologist
Subspecialist in Reproductive Medicine and Surgery
St Mary's Hospital, Central Manchester Foundation Trust
June 2012

Preface

The Part 2 MRCOG is one of the most difficult postgraduate examinations in medicine. The most difficult element is the written papers and many find the MCQs particularly taxing.

Recent changes have included incorporating more MCQs and examiners are setting more evidence-based questions, taken from NICE guidance and RCOG green-top guidelines. We have set out both traditional format MCQs and questions on current guidelines not currently covered in other books. To pass the Part 2 MRCOG MCQ written examination, it is accepted that you must 'practise, practise and practise'!

We have purposely included concise but clear explanatory notes with our answers, particularly on topics that many candidates find difficult. For example, we have devised a series of questions that take the reader through the basic statistical concepts candidates are expected to understand. However, we have strived to maintain both brevity and clarity in our explanations.

The book is primarily intended for candidates sitting the Part 2 MRCOG examination. General practitioner trainees sitting the Diploma of the Royal College of Obstetricians and Gynaecologists examination and medical students may also find this book a useful revision aid.

David J Owen and Muhammad A Akhtar
June 2012

About the authors

David J Owen is nearing the completion of his training and has interests in medical education and psychological medicine. He has worked as a consultant psychiatrist. Dr Owen has recently been nominated for an award for his contribution to undergraduate teaching. His clinical interests are in maternal medicine, intrapartum care, premenstrual syndrome and chronic pelvic pain. He is currently involved in a number of research projects.

Muhammad A Akhtar is a specialty trainee (ST6) in the Mersey Deanery and currently works as senior registrar at University Hospitals Coventry and Warwickshire as out of programme for research (OOPR). He has an interest in reproductive medicine and is currently conducting doctoral research at the University of Warwick. A Cochrane author, in 2012, he updated the 'Progestogens and anti-progestogens for pain associated with endometriosis' review for the Cochrane Database of Systematic Reviews. He is currently writing the 'Heparin for assisted reproduction' review for Cochrane. Dr Akhtar is involved in various research projects and is also an RCOG basic practical skills course facilitator.

Abbreviations

ACN	acute cortical necrosis
AFE	amniotic fluid embolism
AFP	alpha-fetoprotein
AIDS	acquired immune deficiency syndrome
AMH	anti-Müllerian hormone
AVM	arteriovenous malformation
BMI	body mass index
BP	blood pressure
CAH	congenital adrenal hyperplasia
CAIS	complete androgen insensitivity syndrome
CCHB	congenital complete heart block
CF	cystic fibrosis
CHD	congenital heart disease
CMV	*Cytomegalovirus*
COCP	combined oral contraceptive pill
CTG	cardiotocograph
CTPA	computed tomography pulmonary angiogram
DEET	N, N-diethyl-m-toluamide or N, N-diethly-3-methyl-benzamide
DES	diethylstilbestrol
DHEA	dehydroepiandrosterone
DIC	disseminated intravascular coagulation
DMPA	depot medroxyprogesterone acetate
ECV	external cephalic version
EE	ethinylestradiol
EFW	estimated fetal weight
FAI	free androgen index
FIGO	international federation of obstetrics and gynaecology
GBS	Group B Streptococcus
GnRH	gonadotrophin-releasing hormone

HbA$_{1c}$	glycated haemoglobin
HBeAg	hepatitis B 'e' antigen
HBsAg	hepatitis B surface antigen
hCG	human chorionic gonadotrophin
HIV	human immunodeficiency virus
HRT	hormone replacement therapy
HPV	human papillomavirus
HSG	hysterosalpingogram
Ig	immunoglobulin
IUD	intrauterine device
IUGR	intrauterine growth restriction
IUS	intrauterine system
IVC	inferior vena cava
IVF	in vitro fertilisation
LFTs	liver function tests
LMP	last menstrual period
LMWH	low molecular-weight heparin
LNG	levonorgestrel
MCA	middle cerebral artery
MCHC	mean corpuscular haemoglobin concentration
NET-EN	norethisterone enantate
NICE	National Institute for Health and Clinical Excellence
OHSS	ovarian hyperstimulation syndrome
PAPP-A	pregnancy-associated plasma protein A
PCOS	polycystic ovary syndrome
POP	progestogen-only pill
RCT	randomised controlled trial
RDS	respiratory distress syndrome
Rh	Rhesus
RI	resistance index
SAH	subarachnoid haemorrhage
SD	standard deviation
SHBG	sex hormone-binding globulin
SLE	systemic lupus erythematosus
SSRI	selective serotonin reuptake inhibitor
TSH	thyrotropin
TSST-1	toxic shock syndrome toxin 1
TTTS	twin-to-twin transfusion syndrome

UAE	uterine artery embolisation
UDP	uniparental disomy
uE₃	unconjugated oestriol
UKMEC	UK Medical Eligibility Criteria
UPSI	unprotected sexual intercourse
UTI	urinary tract infection
VAIN	vaginal intraepithelial neoplasia
VBAC	vaginal birth after caesarean section
VDRL	Venereal Disease Research Laboratory
VSD	ventricular septal defect
VTE	venous thromboembolism
VZIG	*Varicella zoster* immunoglobulin

This book is dedicated to our life partners for their support, help and encouragement: Fitz and Shumael

The MRCOG written examination comprises 240 MCQ questions set out in two papers, 120 in each paper. These papers are given out at the same time as the EMQ papers, and the RCOG advise that candidates allow 50 minutes for each MCQ paper, i.e. for 120 questions. All questions must be answered true or false. There is no negative marking and therefore every question should be answered. We recommend prospective candidates to visit the RCOG website (www.rcog.org.uk) and read about the examination format well in advance of sitting the written papers. Read each question carefully. Remember MCQs are a test of your knowledge but your scores will improve the more you practise and the more familiar you become with the MCQ format.

1
Obstetrics

Q With regard to the biological effects of ionising radiation on the fetus:
1 stochastic effects are known to have a threshold dose of radiation
2 fetal exposure to radiation doses less than 100 mGy do not result in fetal malformation
3 radiation doses greater than 500 mGy result in severely impaired cognitive function in the fetus.

Q Uniparental disomy (UDP):
4 characteristically occurs sporadically
5 is exemplified by hydatidiform moles and by Prader–Willi syndrome
6 is a reported cause of Angelman syndrome and Beckwith–Wiedemann syndrome.

Q Examples of recessively inherited, single-gene disorders that may be diagnosed prenatally include:
7 Friedreich's ataxia
8 tuberous sclerosis
9 Alport syndrome
10 Duchenne muscular dystrophy
11 sickle cell disease
12 spinal muscular atrophy
13 cystic fibrosis (CF)
14 Tay–Sachs disease
15 Huntington's disease
16 adult polycystic kidney disease
17 thalassaemia
18 Becker muscular dystrophy.

Q In X-linked recessive inheritance:
19 male to male transmission never occurs
20 unaffected males never transmit the disease
21 female homozygotes never occur.

Q The risk of Down's syndrome occurring is:
22 approximately 1% in live-born offspring of female carriers of a Robertsonian 14;21 translocation
23 approximately 10% in live-born offspring of male carriers of a Robertsonian 14;21 translocation.

Q With regard to Klinefelter's syndrome:
  24 the karyotype is 47 XYY
  25 diagnosis is generally made during adult life
  26 when initiated in adolescence, testosterone replacement therapy will improve fertility
  27 there is an increased risk at increased maternal age
  28 there is a recurrence risk of 3%.

Q Each of the following is a recognised association:
  29 Beckwith–Wiedemann syndrome – Wilms' tumour
  30 DiGeorge syndrome – hypoparathyroidism
  31 Turner syndrome – Crohn's disease
  32 trisomy 13 – hypertelorism
  33 trisomy 18 – rocker-bottom feet and short sternum
  34 Apert syndrome – craniosynostosis
  35 Klinefelter's syndrome – diabetes mellitus
  36 Alport syndrome – sensorineural deafness and chronic renal failure
  37 CF – cirrhosis
  38 congenital spherocytosis – spherocytes with decreased mean corpuscular haemoglobin concentration (MCHC)
  39 Gaucher's disease – reduced leukocyte beta-glucocerebrosidase
  40 Marfan's syndrome – lens subluxation
  41 Hurler syndrome – umbilical hernia
  42 osteogenesis imperfecta – blue sclera
  43 myotonic dystrophy – calf pseudohypertrophy
  44 myotonic dystrophy – cataracts
  45 phenylketonuria – congenital heart disease (CHD) and microcephaly
  46 Treacher Collins syndrome – cleft palate
  47 von Hippel–Landau disease – renal carcinoma
  48 neurofibromatosis type I – pheochromocytoma
  49 fetal alcohol syndrome – microcephaly
  50 Noonan syndrome – tall stature.

Q Recognised human teratogens and their associated malformations include:
  51 sodium valproate – hypospadias
  52 thalidomide – phocomelia and anal stenosis
  53 rubella – cataracts.

Q Increased nuchal translucency is associated with:

54 triploidy

55 trisomy 13

56 trisomy 18

57 Fryns syndrome

58 exomphalos

59 diaphragmatic hernia

60 Smith–Lemli–Opitz syndrome.

Q Accurate measurement of nuchal translucency requires:

61 strict coronal view for crown–rump length

62 neutral position of fetal head

63 that the fetus be kept away from amnion

64 the largest of three to five measurements

65 transvaginal scan

66 measurement of maximal distance between fetal skin and cervical vertebra.

Q Each of the following is a change that occurs in the concentration of serum markers associated with Down's syndrome (trisomy 21):

67 pregnancy-associated plasma protein A (PAPP-A) taken in first trimester is decreased

68 human chorionic gonadotrophin (hCG) is decreased

69 alpha-fetoprotein (AFP) is increased

70 inhibin A is increased

71 unconjugated oestriol (uE_3) is decreased.

Q From April 2010, the National Screening Committee has recommended that all maternity units offer women Down's syndrome screening. The screening should provide a detection rate of greater than 90% of affected pregnancies, with a screen-positive rate of less than 2%. Which of the following tests would meet these criteria?

72 measurement of nuchal translucency, hCG and PAPP-A at 11–13 weeks

73 measurement of PAPP-A at 11–13 weeks, then hCG, AFP, uE_3 and inhibin A at 14–20 weeks

74 measurement of nuchal translucency at 11–13 weeks, then PAPP-A, hCG, AFP, uE_3 and inhibin A at 14–20 weeks

75 measurement of hCG, AFP, uE_3 and inhibin A.

Q A 20-week scan for structural abnormalities should detect:

76 80% of major cardiac anomalies

77 90% of diaphragmatic hernia

78 80% of exomphalos or gastroschisis.

Q With regard to fetal blood flow:

79 1% of normal pregnancies have absent end diastolic flow before or at 28 weeks gestation

80 in low-risk pregnancies, studies have demonstrated that more deaths occur in groups allocated to umbilical artery Doppler measurement

81 after 34 weeks in fetuses with growth restriction, the umbilical artery Doppler index may be within the normal range and middle cerebral artery Doppler abnormal, indicating placental cause for intrauterine growth restriction (IUGR)

82 venous Doppler waveforms in umbilical vein, inferior vena cava (IVC) and ductus venosus can be technically difficult to obtain.

Q With regard to cordocentesis in early onset IUGR:

83 there is a 20% chance of fetal bradycardia following cordocentesis

84 pancuronium may be used to paralyse the fetus.

Q Each of the following is a recognised cause of fetal macrosomia:

85 Perlman syndrome

86 MOMO syndrome

87 Marfan's syndrome

88 Weaver–Smith syndrome.

Q Risk factors predisposing to fetal macrosomia include:

89 excessive maternal weight gain

90 female fetus

91 maternal age less than 20 years

92 Hispanic ethnicity.

Q With regard to management of suspected fetal macrosomia:
  93 evidence suggests that inducing labour for suspected fetal macrosomia (estimated fetal weight [EFW] 4.5 kg) increases the rate of caesarean section without improving perinatal outcome
  94 for suspected fetal macrosomia (less than 5 kg) in the absence of maternal diabetes mellitus, prophylactic caesarean section reduces birth trauma significantly
  95 prophylactic caesarean section may be considered when EFW is greater than 5 kg.

Q With regard to fetal cardiac arrhythmias, each of the following is a recognised association:
  96 atrial flutter – Ebstein's malformation
  97 atrial flutter – hydrops fetalis
  98 atrial flutter – maternal (transplacental) digoxin treatment
  99 supraventricular tachycardia – maternal (transplacental) digoxin treatment
  100 sinus bradycardia – long QT interval syndrome
  101 congenital complete heart block (CCHB) – Holt–Oram syndrome.

Q Congenital cardiac heart block (CCHB):
  102 occurs more frequently in women with scleroderma
  103 has a 10%–20% risk for women with anti-Ro and anti-La of having a fetus with complete heart block
  104 has a risk of recurrence in subsequent pregnancy of 10%–15%.

Q With regard to congenital heart disease:
  105 tetralogy of Fallot comprises ventricular septal defect (VSD), overriding aorta, right ventricular outflow obstruction and right ventricular hypertrophy and is associated with DiGeorge syndrome
  106 in addition to causing CHD, 22q11.2 syndrome is associated with learning difficulties, psychiatric illness, cleft palate, facial anomalies and hypertrophic thymus
  107 periconceptual folic acid reduces the risk
  108 most babies with CHD are born to mothers perceived to be at low risk
  109 the risk of CHD is greater in multiple pregnancy
  110 both atrial septal defect and VSD are associated with Down's syndrome

111 risk of recurrence in subsequent pregnancy is greater if the mother rather than the father has CHD

112 patent ductus arteriosus is associated with fetal rubella infection

113 coarctation of aorta is more common in females.

Q Recognised causes of polyhydramnios include:

114 maternal substance misuse

115 lithium therapy

116 sacrococcygeal teratoma

117 congenital syphilis

118 diabetes insipidus

119 renal dysplasia.

Q Maternal complications of polyhydramnios include:

120 post-partum haemorrhage

121 ureteric obstruction

122 higher incidence of pre-eclampsia.

Q Treatment of polyhydramnios includes:

123 sulindac (200 mg twice daily) in gestations greater than 32 weeks

124 amniocentesis in symptomatic women.

Q Recognised causes of oligohydramnios include:

125 posterior urethral valves

126 maternal dehydration

127 diabetes insipidus.

Q Hydrocephalus:

128 is associated with chromosomal abnormality in 1% of cases

129 may be caused by fetal toxoplasmosis

130 is associated with achondroplasia

131 is associated with Dandy–Walker malformation

132 is associated with osteogenesis imperfecta.

Q With regard to neural tube defects:

133 they are associated with Meckel–Gruber syndrome

134 a randomised controlled trial has shown that recurrence rates are reduced significantly by periconceptual folic acid.

Q With regard to microcephaly:
135 in making diagnosis antenatally, measurement of head circumference is preferable to biparietal diameter
136 it is a recognised complication of maternal alcohol misuse.

Q Cases of isolated agenesis of corpus callosum have:
137 a very poor prognosis
138 the pathognomonic ultrasound finding of 'sunburst' lesion.

Q Exomphalos (omphalocele) is associated with:
139 trisomies 13, 18 and 21
140 Beckwith–Wiedemann syndrome
141 triploidy
142 pentalogy of Cantrell
143 Turner syndrome
144 polyhydramnios
145 low levels of maternal serum AFP.

Q With regard to exomphalos:
146 extracorporeal liver is less common than in gastroschisis
147 babies with this should be delivered in a tertiary centre by elective caesarean section.

Q Gastroschisis:
148 is a paraumbilical defect more commonly occurring on the left
149 is sometimes complicated by fetal growth restriction
150 is associated with abnormal karyotype in less than 1% of cases
151 is associated with a higher rate of intrauterine fetal death after 37 weeks
152 may be associated with bowel stenosis.

Q Congenital diaphragmatic hernia is associated with:
153 Fryns syndrome
154 Donnai–Barrow syndrome
155 dextrocardia
156 scaphoid abdomen
157 an antenatal detection rate of 90%
158 poorer prognosis when the liver is present in the thorax
159 polyhydramnios.

Q With regard to oesophageal atresia:

160 it is associated with VACTER syndrome

161 it may be present in DiGeorge syndrome

162 it has an ultrasound appearance of 'double bubble'

163 aneuploidy is present in 10% of cases

164 in isolation, it may be familial.

Q With regard to duodenal atresia:

165 it is associated with annular pancreas

166 approximately 25% of cases have trisomy 21.

Q Jejunal atresia:

167 is associated with apple peel syndrome

168 is strongly associated with trisomy 21

169 may have a recurrence risk of 25% in some cases.

Q Echogenic bowel:

170 is associated with CF in 50% of cases

171 may be transient

172 has increased risk of intrauterine death even in the absence of CF.

Q Echogenic bowel is associated with:

173 aneuploidy

174 *Parvovirus*

175 *Cytomegalovirus* (CMV)

176 meconium ileus

177 intra-amniotic bleeding

178 IUGR

179 polyhydramnios.

Q Congenital cystic adenomatoid malformations:

180 are mostly bilateral

181 derive their blood supply from the aorta

182 are associated with mirror syndrome

183 have a worse prognosis if they cause mediastinal shift.

Q With regard to fetal tumours:
- 184 neuroblastomas are the most common congenital malignant tumours
- 185 sacrococcygeal teratoma is more common in males
- 186 they may originate from maternal metastatic melanoma
- 187 teratomas are the most common congenital brain tumour.

Q With regard to pyelectasis:
- 188 most isolated cases are physiological
- 189 it may be associated with mild reflux
- 190 postnatal evaluation should be performed within 48 hours of delivery.

Q With regard to lower urinary tract obstruction:
- 191 posterior urethral valves are more common in females
- 192 urethral atresia is a lethal abnormality.

Q Prune belly syndrome is:
- 193 associated with undescended testes
- 194 more common in females
- 195 associated with patent urachus
- 196 associated with cocaine misuse.

Q With regard to talipes:
- 197 the most common positional deformity is talipes equinovalgus
- 198 with polyhydramnios, it is suggestive of congenital myotonic dystrophy
- 199 karyotyping is recommended in isolated cases of unilateral talipes equinovarus.

Q Recognised causes of fetal hyperthyroidism include:
- 200 iodine deficiency
- 201 maternal TSH-blocking antibodies
- 202 maternal Hashimoto's thyroiditis
- 203 maternal Graves' disease.

Q Each of the following fetal anomalies is paired with its characteristic ultrasound appearance:

204 agenesis of corpus callosum – 'sunburst' lesion

205 Arnold–Chiari malformation – 'melon' sign

206 posterior urethral valves – 'keyhole' sign

207 jejunal/ileal atresia – 'apple peel' deformity

208 duodenal atresia – 'double bubble' sign.

Q With regard to *Parvovirus* B19 infection:

209 it is characterised by fever, rash ('slapped cheek' and 'lace like' on trunk), arthralgia and anaemia

210 it peaks in late spring and early summer

211 90% of women are immune

212 it is teratogenic in humans

213 it is infectious before onset of symptoms

214 before 20 weeks gestation, risk of fetal loss is 10%

215 after 20 weeks gestation, risk of fetal loss is 5%

216 after 20 weeks gestation, risk of fetal hydrops is 5%

217 hydrops can occur up to 8 weeks after infection

218 spontaneous resolution of hydrops can occur.

Q With regard to CMV:

219 it is the most common cause of non-hereditary deafness

220 it is an RNA virus of the Herpesviridae family

221 it is found in 1% of neonates

222 during primary infection, more fetuses will be infected in the second trimester than in the third trimester

223 the fetus may be infected by exposure to virus in the birth canal.

Q Sequelae of fetal CMV infection include:

224 cataracts

225 hepatosplenomegaly

226 paraventricular cerebral calcification

227 learning disabilities

228 chorioretinitis

229 microcephaly

230 aortic coarctation.

Q With regard to the epidemiology of primary CMV infection:
231 of every 100 women infected, 40 fetuses will become infected, 50% of which will become symptomatic at birth
232 of the asymptomatic infected fetuses, 15% will develop long-term sequelae
233 overall, 20%–25% of infected fetuses will develop long-term sequelae
234 of symptomatic infected fetuses, 20%–30% will die.

Q Congenital rubella causes:
235 cataract
236 intracranial calcification
237 aortic stenosis
238 thrombocytopenia
239 pulmonary artery stenosis
240 patent ductus arteriosus.

Q Listeriosis:
241 is caused by a facultative anaerobic Gram-negative bacillus
242 is uncommon, affecting 12 in 100000 pregnant women
243 is diagnosed by maternal serology
244 causes mid-trimester miscarriage
245 responds well to treatment with intravenous cephalosporins.

Q The clinical features of listeriosis include:
246 backache
247 diarrhoea
248 high neonatal mortality
249 loin pain with concomitant urinary tract infection (UTI)
250 conjunctivitis.

Q Toxoplasmosis:
251 is caused by an obligate intracellular parasite
252 affects 1 in 2000 pregnancies
253 is diagnosed using the Sabin-Feldman dye test, which measures immunoglobulin (Ig) M
254 IgM antibodies for *Toxoplasma gondii* can persist for years after acute infection without any clinical significance.

Q   With regard to toxoplasmosis:
255   90% of maternal infections are asymptomatic
256   when maternal infection is diagnosed, spiramycin should be commenced; the addition of pyrimethamine/sulphadiazine plus folinic acid may be considered if fetal infection is confirmed by polymerase chain reaction of amniotic fluid.

Q   With regard to fetal toxoplasmosis infection:
257   when acquired in the first trimester, there is a greater risk of transmission to the fetus than if acquired in the third trimester
258   acute maternal infection in the third trimester is associated with transmission to the fetus in 60% of cases.

Q   Fetal toxoplasmosis causes:
259   intracerebral calcification
260   hydrocephalus
261   microcephaly
262   chorioretinitis
263   ascites
264   thrombocytopenia.

Q   With regard to subarachnoid haemorrhage (SAH) occurring in pregnancy:
265   the greatest risk is during the third trimester
266   most cases are due to rupture of arterial (berry) aneurysm
267   it is a common cause of indirect maternal death
268   when caused by ruptured berry aneurysm, it is most likely to occur during labour.

Q   With regard to migraine in pregnancy:
269   most migraineurs experience improvement during their pregnancy
270   it may be treated prophylactically with aspirin (75 mg daily), beta-blockers and tricyclic antidepressants
271   pizotifen is absolutely contraindicated
272   ergotamine is absolutely contraindicated.

Q   Clinical features of cerebral vein thrombosis may include:
273   fever with leukocytosis
274   photophobia.

Q Benign intracranial hypertension:

275 tends to occur in obese women over the age of 35 years

276 tends to improve during pregnancy

277 when new onset, most often presents during the second trimester

278 may be treated with acetazolamide

279 may cause blindness due to optic nerve infarction.

Q Bell's palsy:

280 occurs more commonly during pregnancy and most frequently peripartum

281 typically involves bilateral lower motor neurone lesion of the facial nerve

282 may be associated with loss of taste on the posterior two-thirds of the tongue

283 characteristically results in absent corneal reflex and inability to produce tears on affected side.

Q Carpal tunnel syndrome is:

284 caused by compression of the median nerve and is characteristically associated with Cullen's sign

285 more common in women with hypothyroidism.

Q In pregnant women with myasthenia gravis:

286 magnesium sulphate should be avoided as it may precipitate a crisis

287 salbutamol may worsen symptoms

288 epidural anaesthesia is relatively contraindicated

289 neonatal myasthenia gravis is common (20%) and occurs in the first 2 days following birth

290 the first stage of labour is usually prolonged.

Q Myotonic dystrophy is associated with increased risk of:

291 polyhydramnios

292 preterm delivery

293 placental praevia

294 post-partum haemorrhage

295 stillbirth

296 regional anaesthetic complications.

Q With regard to multiple sclerosis, during pregnancy:

297 women are more likely to suffer relapse

298 UTIs occur more commonly

Q Recognised teratogenic effects of anti-epileptic drugs include:

299 hypertelorism

300 hypoplastic nails

301 low-set ears.

Q With regard to epilepsy, the risk of seizures in pregnancy is increased by:

302 labour

303 anxiety

304 pain.

Q With regard to obstetric cholestasis:

305 it tends to occur earlier in women with hepatitis C infection

306 it has a recurrence rate of 90%

307 the bilirubin level is typically raised

308 a normal level of serum bile acids excludes diagnosis.

Q With regard to severe asthma in pregnancy:

309 prostaglandin E_2 is contraindicated

310 leukotriene antagonists should be stopped pre-pregnancy

311 acute attacks may be exacerbated by intravenous magnesium sulphate

Q Each of the following drugs used to treat tuberculosis is matched with its recognised side effect:

312 rifampicin – orange secretions

313 isoniazid – peripheral neuropathy

314 streptomycin – fetal 7th cranial nerve damage

315 ethambutol – peripheral neuropathy.

Q Sarcoidosis in pregnancy is associated with:

316 hypoparathyroidism in the neonate

317 neonatal tetany at birth.

Q With regard to CF in pregnancy:
318 diabetes mellitus is more common
319 it is associated with reduced fertility
320 all women should be screened for diabetes.

Q Women with sickle cell trait (HbAS) are more prone to:
321 UTI in pregnancy
322 pre-eclampsia.

Q Women with sickle cell disease (HbSS) are at greater risk of:
323 bone marrow embolism
324 streptococcal infection
325 pre-eclampsia
326 preterm delivery
327 sickling crises during pregnancy
328 requiring blood transfusion.

Q Women with HbSC disease:
329 are at higher risk of anaemia

Q In sickle cell (HbSS) disease in pregnancy:
330 mean corpuscular haemoglobin is typically normal
331 haemoglobin S has a lower affinity for oxygen than haemoglobin A
332 splenomegaly often occurs
333 hyposplenism is common
334 folate deficiency is common
335 there is an increased incidence of red blood cell antibodies.

Q Recognised complications of sickle cell (HbSS) disease in pregnancy include:
336 cholelithiasis and acute cholecystitis
337 bone marrow suppression
338 fat emboli
339 seizures
340 splenic sequestration
341 pre-eclampsia
342 cerebral abscess
343 subarachnoid haemorrhage.

Q With regard to thalassaemia syndromes:

344 beta-thalassaemia major is incompatible with life

345 alpha-thalassaemia major sufferers are at increased risk of requiring caesarean section

346 parenteral iron should be given when ferritin levels are low

347 iron chelation therapy (desferioxamine) should be stopped during pregnancy.

Q Recognised causes of maternal thrombocytopenia include:

348 hepatic vein thrombosis

349 portal hypertension

350 systemic lupus erythematosus (SLE)

351 splenectomy

352 amniotic fluid embolism

353 deficiency of von Willebrand factor (vWf)-cleaving protease.

Q With regard to acute fatty liver of pregnancy:

354 it is more common in women carrying a male fetus

355 it is more common in obese women

356 it is associated with diabetes insipidus

357 it is associated with profound hypoglycaemia

358 liver biopsy demonstrates microvesicular fatty infiltration of hepatocytes periportally with central sparing and marked necrosis

Q Clinical features of mitral stenosis may include:

359 pulmonary oedema

360 haemoptysis

361 atrial flutter

362 atrial fibrillation and pulmonary hypotension

363 malar flush

364 low-pitched mid-systolic murmur

365 loud first heart sound

366 'opening snap'.

Q Peripartum cardiomyopathy:
367 typically occurs in the second or third trimester
368 causes cerebral embolism
369 causes coronary embolism
370 is associated with superior mesenteric artery occlusion
371 may be treated by cardiac transplant
372 has a recurrence rate of 50% in subsequent pregnancy

Q Hyperemesis gravidarum is a recognised cause of:
373 central pontine myelinolysis secondary to vitamin B1 deficiency
374 spastic quadriparesis
375 Korsakoff's psychosis
376 metabolic hypochloraemic acidosis.

Q With regard to asymptomatic bacteria in pregnancy:
377 5% of pregnant women in the UK will be affected, of whom 90% will develop symptomatic UTI
378 treatment reduces risk of preterm delivery and low birth weight.

Q With regard to renal disease in pregnancy:
379 women with pre-eclampsia are at greater risk of developing renal cortical necrosis
380 haemolytic uraemic syndrome is commonly associated with hypertension.

Q With regard to pre-existing diabetes during pregnancy:
381 proliferative retinopathy has a 50% chance of worsening
382 the presence of microvascular disease increases the risk of developing hypertension
383 instituting a strict regimen of glycaemic control decreases the risk of deterioration of non-proliferative retinopathy
384 for every 1% reduction in glycated haemoglobin (HbA_{1c}) during the first 20 weeks of pregnancy, there is a significant increase in episodes of hypoglycaemia.

Q With regard to SLE:

385 it is more common in Afro-Caribbean women

386 there is an increased risk of flares during pregnancy

387 the risk of adverse pregnancy outcome is higher in women if SLE is active periconceptually

388 there is an anti-nuclear antibody titre increase during disease activity.

Q The following drugs are correctly matched to their side effect/adverse event:

389 methyldopa – bradycardia

390 hydralazine – erythema multiforme

391 nifedipine – palpitations

392 oxytocin – hypernatraemia

393 mifepristone – exacerbation of severe asthma

394 atosiban – hyperglycaemia

395 terbutaline – hypotension

396 ergometrine – myocardial infarction.

Q When used to prevent pre-eclampsia, the benefits of antenatal low dose aspirin (75 mg daily) include:

397 reduction in the risk of pre-eclampsia

398 reduction in preterm delivery

399 reduction in IUGR

400 reduction in the risk of placental abruption

401 overall reduction of the incidence of pregnancy-induced hypertension

402 reduction in stillbirth.

Q Recognised risk factors for placental abruption include:

403 bilateral notching on umbilical artery

404 raised second-trimester AFP

405 external cephalic version (ECV).

Q There is an increased risk of placenta praevia in:

406 women with a history of miscarriage

407 smokers

408 cocaine users.

Q   Factors known to predispose to breech presentation include:
409   hydrocephalus
410   Prader–Willi syndrome
411   cornual placenta
412   maternal alcohol misuse.

Q   The incidence of monozygotic twins is higher among:
413   African women
414   older women
415   women undergoing in vitro fertilisation (IVF).

Q   With regard to twins:
416   30% are monozygotic
417   30% of monozygotic twins are dichorionic diamniotic
418   twin-to-twin transfusion syndrome (TTTS) never occurs in monoamniotic twins

Q   With regard to TTTS:
419   unidirectional arterio-arterial anastomoses are thought to be causal
420   the recipient twin in Quintero stage II becomes the 'stuck twin'
421   compared with amniodrainage, laser coagulation has been shown to improve neurological outcome as measured at 6 months

Q   With regard to vaginal breech delivery:
422   the Term Breech Trial (2000) has demonstrated 100 caesarean sections are needed to prevent one perinatal death
423   there is insufficient evidence to justify caesarean section for preterm singleton breeches.

Q   Risk factors associated with unstable lie include:
424   large ovarian cyst
425   uterine malformation
426   macrosomia
427   placenta praevia.

Q Face presentation is:

428 more common in preterm labour

429 associated with meningocele

430 associated with anencephaly

431 associated with fetal goitre.

Q The following malpositions are correctly paired with their sagittal diameter of fetal head:

432 brow presentation – submentobregmatic

433 face presentation – mentovertical

434 occipito-posterior presentation – occipitobregmatic.

Q With regard to intrauterine fetal death:

435 the stillbirth rate is the number of stillbirths per 1000 live births plus stillbirths

436 the perimortality rate is the number of stillborn and neonatal deaths per 1000 live births plus stillbirths.

Q Increased risk of intrauterine death occurs with:

437 maternal age less than 20 years

438 inherited thrombophilias

439 group B streptococcal infection

440 maternal thyrotoxicosis.

Q In a water birth:

441 the water temperature should be 37°C

442 immersion should only take place when the cervix is dilated 5 cm or more

443 the fetal heart rate should be monitored using an underwater Doppler device

444 the woman should not return to the pool if she gets out during the second stage.

Q With regard to epidural anaesthesia in labour:

445 the epidural space is entered at L2–L5

446 there is an increased risk of operative vaginal delivery

447 it is contraindicated in women taking aspirin

448 dural taps can be treated by introducing an autologous blood patch which has a success rate of 50%.

Q According to the National Institute for Health and Clinical Excellence (NICE) guidelines (2008) on induction of labour:

449 vaginal prostaglandin (E_2) should be used in preference to oxytocin in nulliparous and parous women with intact membranes, regardless of their cervical favourability.

Q With regard to fetal electronic monitoring:

450 fetal heart rate patterns demonstrating complicated baseline tachycardia are more likely to be associated with fetal acidosis than uncomplicated loss of baseline variability

451 it has been shown to significantly reduce the incidence of neonatal seizures.

Q With amniotic fluid embolism (AFE):

452 most cases occur during caesarean section

453 most AFEs occur within 3 minutes of amniotomy

454 most deaths occur rapidly after the acute event

455 the presence of squamous cells in the pulmonary circulation is diagnostic.

Q Each of the following is a risk factor for post-partum haemorrhage:

456 maternal age greater than 35 years

457 Asian ethnicity

458 anaemia

459 physiological third stage

460 pyrexia in labour.

Q At risk for developing disseminated intravascular coagulation (DIC) in pregnancy are those with:

461 acute fatty liver of pregnancy

462 hydatidiform mole

463 placenta praevia.

Q The causes of neonatal jaundice appearing on the third day and persisting for 14 days include:

464 galactosaemia

465 haemolysis due to Rhesus (Rh) incompatibility

466 neonatal hypothyroidism

467 biliary atresia

468 glucose-6-phosphate dehydrogenase deficiency.

Q The causes of neonatal jaundice appearing in the first 24 hours include:

469 Rh incompatibility

470 ABO incompatibility

471 glucose-6-phosphate dehydrogenase deficiency

472 congenital spherocytosis.

Q Thromboprophylaxis after delivery in women with sickle cell disease includes low molecular-weight heparin (LMWH):

473 administered for 3 days following vaginal delivery

474 administered for 7 days following caesarean section

Q In the intrapartum management of sickle cell disease in pregnancy:

475 regional anaesthesia should be avoided

476 pethidine should be avoided

477 morphine should be avoided

478 pregnant women with healthy well-grown fetuses should be offered elective induction of labour or caesarean delivery at 40 + 0 weeks.

Q Regarding the preconceptual management of women with sickle cell disease:

479 5 mg folic acid should be taken daily

480 hydroxyurea should be stopped 6 months prior to conception

481 echocardiography should be used to screen for pulmonary hypertension

482 retinal screening should be performed to detect proliferative retinopathy.

Q The following vaccines should be given to or updated in women with sickle cell disease prior to achieving pregnancy:

483 *Haemophilus influenzae* type B

484 meningococcal C

485 hepatitis B

486 pneumococcal

487 influenza.

Q Amniocentesis:
488 should be performed from 14 weeks onwards
489 has a 1% risk of miscarriage
490 may cause fetal talipes
491 requires an outer needle with a maximum size of 18 gauge
492 in the third trimester appears to be associated with emergency delivery
493 mid-trimester more commonly requires multiple attempts
494 in the third trimester more commonly has blood-stained fluid.

Q Chorionic villus sampling:
495 should be performed only by transabdominal approach
496 should not be performed before 10 completed weeks of gestation
497 is associated with limb reduction defects
498 is associated with oromandibular hypoplasia
499 can be technically difficult to perform before 11 weeks.

Q Antenatal steroids are associated with a significant reduction in the rate of:
500 neonatal death by 31%
501 respiratory distress syndrome by 44%
502 intraventricular haemorrhage by 46%.

Q Antenatal corticosteroid use is associated with reduction in fetal:
503 necrotising enterocolitis
504 intensive care admissions
505 systemic infections in the first 48 hours of life.

Q Regarding antenatal corticosteroids:
506 these are most effective in reducing respiratory distress syndrome (RDS) in pregnancies that deliver within 24 hours and up to 7 days after administration of the second dose
507 there is a significant higher risk of cerebral palsy among children who have been exposed to repeated doses of corticosteroids
508 repeated doses are associated with small for gestational age at birth
509 multiple doses are associated with smaller head circumference
510 should be given to all women for whom an elective caesarean section is planned prior to 38 + 0 weeks of gestation.

Q Infants exposed to antenatal betamethasone rather than antenatal dexamethasone:

511 have less neonatal cystic periventricular leukomalacia

512 have a similar rate of neonatal death

513 have a greater reduction in RDS.

Q Each of the following factors is associated with unsuccessful vaginal birth after caesarean section (VBAC):

514 previous vaginal birth

515 induced labour

516 body mass index (BMI) greater than 30

517 VBAC at or after 41 weeks of gestation

518 epidural anaesthesia

519 non-white ethnicity

520 previous preterm caesarean birth

521 more than 2 years since previous caesarean birth

522 advanced maternal age

523 female fetus.

Q Risk of uterine rupture in:

524 unscarred uterus is 2 per 10 000

525 previous high vertical classical caesarean section is 200–900 per 10 000

526 prior inverted T or J incision is 190 per 10 000

527 previous low transverse caesarean section and spontaneous labour is 22 per 10 000

528 previous low transverse caesarean section and syntocinon augmentation is 87 per 10 000

529 previous low transverse caesarean section and prostaglandin induction of labour is 102 per 10 000.

Q There is statistically significant risk of the following associated with vaginal birth after caesarean section compared with elective repeat caesarean section:

530 blood transfusion

531 endometritis

532 hysterectomy

533 thromboembolic disease

534 maternal death.

Q Clinical features that may be indicative of uterine rupture include:

535 abnormal CTG

536 abdominal pain persisting between contractions

537 chest pain

538 sudden onset of shortness of breath

539 haematuria

540 cessation of uterine activity

541 maternal bradycardia.

Q Regarding blood transfusion:

542 patient blood samples used for cross-matching red cells should be no more than 5 days old

543 anti-c in pregnancy is more likely to have been induced by previous transfusion

544 anti-K in pregnancy is more likely to have been induced by previous transfusion

545 in pregnancy, pre-autologous deposit can be used.

Q Kell-negative blood should be used for transfusion in women of childbearing age due to high risk of:

546 alloimmunisation

547 subsequent haemolytic disease of the newborn.

Q Cell salvage in pregnancy:

548 is recommended for women in whom an intraoperative blood loss of more than 1000 mL is anticipated

549 does not necessarily require the patient's consent.

Q Anti-D prophylaxis is not required if an Rh D-negative woman receives:

550 Rh D-positive fresh frozen plasma (FFP)

551 Rh D-positive cryoprecipitate.

Q With regard to platelet transfusion:

552 Rh D-negative women should receive Rh D-negative platelets

553 it should be group compatible ideally.

Q Incidence of breech presentation is:
554 40% at 28 weeks of gestation
555 5%–6% at term.

Q Unfavourable factors for successful vaginal breech birth include:
556 frank breech
557 footling breech
558 baby weighing more than 3500 g
559 small-for-gestational-age baby
560 previous caesarean section.

Q With regard to primary *Varicella zoster* infection:
561 it is characterised by a pruritic maculopapular rash
562 it has an incubation period of 1–3 weeks
563 it is infectious 48 hours before the rash appears and continues to be infectious until the vesicles crust over within 5 days
564 it has an incidence of 3/1000 pregnancies
565 risk of miscarriage is increased if chicken pox is developed in the first trimester
566 risk of severe neonatal infection is greatest when rash onset is 5 days before and up to 2 days after delivery.

Q *V. zoster* vaccine:
567 contains live attenuated virus
568 is derived from the Oka strain of *V. zoster* virus.

Q With regard to *Varicella zoster* immunoglobulin (VZIG):
569 pregnant women are potentially infectious from 8 to 28 days after VZIG is given
570 pregnant women are potentially infectious from 8 to 21 days if no VZIG is given
571 a second dose of VZIG may be required if a further exposure is reported and 3 weeks have elapsed since the last dose
572 VZIG has some therapeutic benefit once chickenpox has developed.

Q Fetal varicella syndrome may include:
573 chorioretinitis
574 cataracts

575 hypoplasia of the limbs

576 hydrocephaly

577 dysfunction of bowel sphincters

578 dysfunction of bladder sphincters.

Q External cephalic version (ECV):

579 is offered from 37 weeks in nulliparous women

580 is offered from 36 weeks in multiparous women

581 appears to promote labour

582 can cause fetal tachycardia

583 can cause a nonreactive CTG

584 can cause alterations in uterine artery waveform

585 can result in an increase in amniotic fluid volume.

Q Relative contraindications for ECV include:

586 small-for-gestational-age fetus with abnormal Doppler parameters

587 ruptured membranes

588 oligohydramnios

589 major fetal anomalies

590 one previous caesarean section.

Q Acute complications of female genital mutilation include:

591 tetanus

592 retention of urine

593 hepatitis

594 human immunodeficiency virus (HIV)

595 death

596 sexual dysfunction

597 haematocolpos

598 implantation dermoid cysts.

Q Incidence of:

599 neonatal herpes is annually 1/60 000 live births

600 early onset Group B streptococcal (GBS) neonatal infection is 1/10 000 births

601 sudden infant death is 1/10 000 live births

602 maternal mortality in the UK is 14/100 000 births.

Q Mortality from early onset GBS neonatal sepsis in the UK is:

603 9% in term infants

604 18% in preterm infants.

Q To prevent one neonatal death from early onset GBS neonatal sepsis:

605 7000 colonised women need to be given intrapartum antibiotic prophylaxis

606 24000 women need to be screened.

Q Breastfeeding increases the risk of:

607 neonatal GBS

608 HIV transmission.

Q Regarding HIV testing in pregnancy:

609 third-generation laboratory assays are recommended as the first-line HIV test for antenatal screening

610 in women booking for antenatal care at or after 26 weeks, the test should be requested urgently and the result issued within 24 hours

611 during the antenatal booking visit, all women who are HIV positive should be checked to ensure they are having yearly cervical cytology.

Q Each of the following immunisations can be administered safely in pregnancy:

612 hepatitis B

613 pneumococcus

614 influenza

615 *V. zoster*

616 measles.

Q In all neonates born to women who are HIV positive:

617 antiretroviral therapy should be commenced within 6 hours of birth

618 tests should be performed at 1 day, 6 weeks and 12 weeks of age

619 if all previous tests are negative, a confirmatory HIV antibody test should be performed at around 18 months of age.

Q Infections associated with stillbirths include:

620 CMV

621 syphilis

622 *Parvovirus* B19

623 *Listeria*

624 *Rubella*

625 toxoplasmosis

626 *Herpes simplex*

627 coxsackievirus

628 *Leptospira*

629 Q fever

630 Lyme disease

631 malaria.

Q Regarding stillbirth:

632 6% of stillborn babies will have a chromosomal abnormality

633 more than 85% of women with intrauterine fetal death could labour spontaneously within 3 weeks of diagnosis

634 there is a 10% chance of maternal DIC within 4 weeks of the date of fetal death.

Q DNA-based methods for routine chromosome analysis are superior to cell culture because:

635 the failure rate is 1%

636 they are cost-effective techniques for detecting common aneuploidies

637 they are reliable for the detection of translocations

638 they are reliable for detection of marker chromosomes.

Q Regarding perinatal specimens suitable for karyotyping:

639 skin specimens are associated with a higher rate of culture failure

640 placental tissue can show pseudomosaicism

641 cartilage from the patella can be used for karyotyping.

Q Regarding suppression of lactation:

642 cabergoline is superior to bromocriptine

643 dopamine agonists should not be given to women with hypertension.

Q Pregnancy affected with malaria can result in:

644 miscarriage

645 stillbirth

646 prematurity

647 fetal anaemia

648 low birth weight.

Q Clinical findings of severe malaria in adults include:

649 pulmonary oedema

650 convulsions

651 jaundice

652 haemoglobinuria.

Q Laboratory test results in severe malaria show:

653 thrombocytosis

654 hypoglycaemia

655 acidosis (pH < 7.3)

656 hyperlactataemia.

Q Regarding malaria in pregnancy:

657 *Plasmodium falciparum* malaria is more severe than any other form of malaria

658 for diagnosis in pregnancy, rapid diagnostic tests to detect specific parasite antigens or enzymes are less sensitive than thick and thin malaria blood films

659 fatality in uncomplicated *P. falciparum* malaria is 5%

660 fatality in complicated severe malaria is 15%–20% in non-pregnant women

661 fatality in complicated severe malaria is 50% in pregnant women

662 non-*falciparum* species are rarely fatal

663 treatments in pregnancy may have lower efficacy than in non-pregnant patients.

Q The following medications can be used in the treatment of malaria in pregnancy:
664 artesunate in severe *falciparum* malaria
665 quinine and clindamycin to treat uncomplicated *P. falciparum*
666 quinine and clindamycin to treat uncomplicated mixed *P. falciparum*, *Plasmodium vivax*
667 chloroquine to treat *P. vivax*, *Plasmodium ovale* or *Plasmodium malariae*
668 primaquine to treat *P. vivax*, *P. ovale* or *P. malariae*.

Q Side effects of quinine include:
669 tinnitus
670 headache
671 altered auditory acuity
672 blurred vision
673 vertigo.

Q Regarding prophylaxis of malaria in pregnancy:
674 20% DEET (N, N-diethyl-m-toluamide or N, N-diethly-3-methyl-benzamide) solution is safe to use in the second and third trimesters of pregnancy
675 20% DEET solution can be found in cord blood
676 mefloquine (5 mg/kg once per week) is the recommended drug of choice for prophylaxis in the second and third trimesters in chloroquine-resistant areas.

Q Twin-to-twin transfusion syndrome (TTTS):
677 complicates 25% of monochorionic pregnancies
678 is more common in monochorionic, diamniotic than monochorionic, monoamniotic pregnancies
679 reverse transfusion can occur in 1% of cases
680 commonly involves velamentous cord insertions
681 presenting severely before 26 weeks of gestation should be treated by amnioreduction or septostomy
682 can recur later in 14% of pregnancies treated by laser ablation.

Q Obstetric cholestasis:
683 affects 0.7% of pregnancies in multi-ethnic populations
684 affects 1.5% of women of Indian-Asian or Pakistani Asian origin
685 once obstetric cholestasis is diagnosed, it is reasonable to perform liver function tests (LFTs) twice weekly
686 postnatal LFTs should be deferred for at least 7 days.

Q Obstetric cholestasis is associated with:
687 premature birth
688 meconium-stained liquor
689 higher rates of caesarean section
690 post-partum haemorrhage.

Q Each of the following interventions reduces the incidence of assisted vaginal delivery:
691 continuous support for women during labour
692 an upright position in the second stage of labour
693 a lateral position in the second stage of labour
694 a supine position in the second stage of labour
695 the lithotomy position in the second stage of labour
696 epidural analgesia.

Q Each of the following is an indication for operative vaginal delivery:
697 maternal cardiac disease class II
698 myasthenia gravis
699 proliferative retinopathy
700 lack of continuing progress for 2 hours (active and passive second stage) in a nulliparous woman.

Q Compared with forceps, vacuum extraction is less likely to:
701 fail
702 be associated with retinal haemorrhage
703 be associated with maternal worries about baby
704 cause significant maternal perineal trauma
705 require that phototherapy be used for the neonate.

Q Risk of intracranial haemorrhage in the neonate:
706 is 1/256 operative vaginal deliveries when two instruments are used
707 is 1/334 deliveries when 'failed forceps' delivery proceeds to caesarean section.

Q Vasa praevia:
708 is described as fetal vessels coursing through the membranes over the external cervical os and below the fetal presenting part, unprotected by placental tissue or the umbilical cord
709 is associated with velamentous cord insertion
710 is not associated with accessory lobes of placenta
711 incidence is 1/2000–6000 pregnancies
712 carries no major maternal risk.

Q Risk factors for vasa praevia include:
713 succenturiate lobes of placenta
714 multiple pregnancies
715 IVF.

Q Risk factors for post-partum haemorrhage include:
716 Asian ethnicity
717 BMI greater than 35
718 pyrexia in labour
719 age greater than 40 years.

Q Risk factors for breast cancer include:
720 nulliparity
721 early menarche
722 young age at first pregnancy.

Q Tocolytic drugs to prevent preterm labour are not associated with a clear reduction in:
723 perinatal mortality and morbidity
724 neonatal mortality and morbidity.

Q Preterm premature rupture of the membranes:
725 complicates 2% of pregnancies
726 is associated with 40% of preterm deliveries.

Q Regarding fetal movements:

727 the number of spontaneous movements tends to increase until the twenty-eighth week of pregnancy

728 the type of fetal movement may change as pregnancy advances in the third trimester

729 by term, the average number of generalised movements per hour is 10

730 the longest period between fetal movements ranges from 50 to 75 minutes

731 peak fetal activity occurs in the evening and night-time

732 fetal presentation has an effect on perception of movement

733 approximately 90% of women who perceive a reduction in fetal movements will have a normal outcome to their pregnancy.

Q Regarding the findings of The MAGPIE study, it is incorrect that:

734 women allocated magnesium sulphate rather than placebo had a 58% lower risk of an eclampsia

735 maternal mortality was lower in the magnesium sulphate group

736 magnesium sulphate reduced the risk of placental abruption

737 if magnesium sulphate is given, it should be continued for 24 hours following delivery or 24 hours after the last seizure.

Q Shoulder dystocia:

738 could be caused by posterior fetal shoulder

739 has an incidence of 0.6%.

Q Factors associated with shoulder dystocia include:

740 prolonged first stage of labour

741 oxytocin augmentation.

Q Risk factors for third-degree perineal tears include:

742 occipito-posterior position

743 multiparity

744 epidural analgesia

745 mediolateral episiotomy.

Q Regarding thromboprophylaxis:

746 women with previous thromboses and antiphospholipid syndrome should be offered both antenatal and 6 weeks of post-partum thromboprophylaxis

747 women with persistent antiphospholipid antibodies with no previous venous thromboembolism (VTE) and no other risk factors may be managed with close surveillance antenatally but should be considered for 7 days of post-partum thromboprophylaxis

748 women with asymptomatic inherited thrombophilia without other risk factors may be managed with close surveillance antenatally but should be considered for 7 days of post-partum thromboprophylaxis

749 women with antithrombin deficiency or more than one thrombophilic defect (including homozygous factor V Leiden, homozygous prothrombin G20210A and compound heterozygotes) should have antenatal and postnatal thromboprophylaxis

750 women with previous thromboses and antiphospholipid syndrome should be offered both antenatal and 6 weeks of post-partum thromboprophylaxis.

Q Risk of epidural haematoma can be avoided if:

751 regional techniques are not used until at least 6 hours after the previous prophylactic dose of LMWH

752 regional techniques are not used for at least 12 hours after the last therapeutic dose of LMWH

753 the thromboprophylactic dose of LMWH is given 4 hours post-operatively

754 the thromboprophylactic dose of LMWH is not given until 4 hours after the epidural catheter has been removed.

Q Danaparoid:

755 is only administered by subcutaneous injection

756 has both anti-IIa and anti-Xa effects

757 has a long anti-Xa effect

758 has a half-life of about 12 hours

759 use can result in anti-Xa activity in the breast milk of women

760 use can result in anti-factor Xa activity in the umbilical cord plasma of newborn babies.

Q Fondaparinux:
761 is a synthetic disaccharide
762 functions as an anticoagulant
763 is licensed in the UK for the prevention and treatment of VTE outside pregnancy
764 has a broadly similar efficacy to LMWH
765 use can result in anti-factor Xa activity in the umbilical cord plasma.

Q Lepirudin:
766 is an anticoagulant
767 crosses the placenta.

Q Graduated compression stockings of appropriate strength are recommended in pregnancy and the puerperium for women:
768 who are hospitalised and have a contraindication to LMWH
769 travelling long distance for more than 4 hours.

Q The following statements are correct:
770 a ventilation perfusion scan has a risk of childhood cancer similar to that of a computed tomography pulmonary angiogram (CTPA)
771 the lifetime risk of maternal breast cancer is increased by up to 13% with CTPA
772 routine platelet count monitoring should not be carried out with LMWH
773 graduated elastic compression stockings should be worn on the affected leg for 1 year after the acute event to reduce the risk of post-thrombotic syndrome
774 post-thrombotic syndrome following deep vein thrombosis is found in over 60% of cases.

Q Risk factors for cord prolapse include:
775 being nulliparous
776 birth weight less than 2.5 kg
777 ECV procedure
778 low-lying placenta.

Q The rate of complications for performed caesarean sections during labour:
779 at 0–1 cm cervical dilatation is 17/100
780 at 9–10 cm dilatation is 33/100.

Q With caesarean section, the risk of:
781 emergency hysterectomy is 1/1000
782 admission to intensive care unit is 5/1000
783 thromboembolic disease is 4–16/1000
784 bladder injury is 1/1000
785 ureteric injury is 3/10 000
786 death is 1/12 000
787 antepartum stillbirth in future pregnancy is 1–4/1000
788 placenta praevia, including placenta accrete in future pregnancy is 4–8/1000
789 readmission to hospital is 5/1000
790 haemorrhage is 5/1000
791 infection is 6/100
792 fetal lacerations is 2/100.

Q With caesarean section for placenta praevia, the risk of:
793 emergency hysterectomy is 7/100
794 need for further laparotomy during recovery is 7/100
795 future placenta praevia is 23/1000.

Q With the repair of third- and fourth-degree tears, the risk of:
796 faecal urgency is 9/100
797 perineal pain is 9/100
798 dyspareunia is 9/100
799 wound infection is 8/100.

Q Cord blood is used in the treatment of:
800 leukaemia
801 sickle cell anaemia
802 Hurler syndrome.

Q With regard to cord blood transplants:
803 they have fewer complications than bone marrow transplants
804 they are more difficult than bone marrow transplants to find stem cell matches for
805 cord blood can be frozen and stored for years, whereas bone marrow cannot.

Q According to NICE guidelines (intrapartum care, 2007), during the first stage of labour:

806 fetal heart rate should be checked every 15 minutes after a contraction

807 the frequency of contractions should be documented every 15 minutes

808 pulse should be checked every 4 hours

809 maternal blood pressure (BP) and temperature should be checked every 4 hours.

Q According to NICE guidelines (intrapartum care, 2007), during the second stage of labour:

810 fetal heart rate should be checked every 5 minutes after a contraction

811 the frequency of contractions should be documented every 15 minutes

812 pulse should be checked every 30 minutes

813 BP and temperature should be checked every hour

814 the woman should be discouraged from lying supine/semi-supine.

Q Regarding smoking:

815 a carbon monoxide (CO) test is an immediate, non-invasive biochemical method for assessing whether someone smokes

816 motivational interviewing is effective in helping pregnant women to quit smoking.

Q Regarding antidepressant use during pregnancy:

817 most tricyclic antidepressants have a higher fatal toxicity index than selective serotonin reuptake inhibitors (SSRIs)

818 fluoxetine is the SSRI with the lowest known risk during pregnancy

819 SSRIs taken after 20 weeks' gestation are associated with an increased risk of persistent pulmonary hypertension in the neonate

820 paroxetine taken in the first trimester is associated with fetal heart defects

821 venlafaxine is associated with an increased risk of high BP.

Q With regard to drugs used in pregnancy:

822 antidepressants can be prescribed for the short-term treatment of extreme anxiety and agitation

823 benzodiazepines are associated with cleft palate in the fetus

824 clozapine causes agranulocytosis in the fetus

825 lamotrigine is associated with Stevens–Johnson syndrome in infants

826 olanzapine is associated with gestational diabetes and weight loss.

Q For women who have had pre-eclampsia, in a future pregnancy:

827 the risk of developing gestational hypertension is up to 1/5 pregnancies

828 the risk of developing pre-eclampsia is up to approximately 1/10 pregnancies.

Q Breastfeeding is safe with this anti-hypertensive medication:

829 enalapril

830 captopril

831 atenolol

832 metoprolol.

Q The level of this antidepressant present is high in breast milk:

833 imipramine

834 sertraline

835 citalopram

836 fluoxetine.

2
Gynaecology

Q Congenital adrenal hyperplasia (CAH):

1 may be associated with ambiguous genitalia

2 can present later in childhood

3 can be associated with absent aldosterone

4 delayed diagnosis may result in short stature

5 displays sex-linked inheritance

6 is caused by 11-hydroxylase deficiency

7 is caused by 3 beta-hydroxysteroid dehydrogenase deficiency

8 is caused by 21-hydroxylase deficiency in a minority of cases

9 may cause vaginal stenosis.

Q Complete vaginal agenesis:

10 occurs in approximately 75% of cases of Mayer–Rokitansky–Küster–Hauser syndrome

11 may occur in androgen insensitivity syndrome

12 is commonly found in CAH

13 is commonly associated with urological abnormalities.

Q Prepubertal vulvovaginitis may be caused by:

14 Kawasaki disease

15 *Enterobius vermicularis*

16 ectopic ureter

17 scarlet fever

18 mononucleosis

19 candidiasis.

Q Prepubertal labial adhesions:

20 should be treated with topical oestrogen

21 occurring after the age of 4 years may indicate sexual abuse

22 may present with bleeding.

Q Regarding ovarian neoplasms in childhood and adolescence:

23 the most common is the benign cystic teratoma (dermoid)

24 the most common are germ cell tumours

25 dysgerminoma is benign and occurs bilaterally in 15% of cases

26 endodermal sinus tumours are rare.

Q Dermoid cysts (benign cystic teratomas):

27 are the most common sex cord-stromal ovarian tumours

28 account for 60% of all ovarian neoplasms

29 have the risk of malignant transformation, which is greater in prepubescent girls

30 are bilateral in 10%–15% of cases

31 may transform into squamous cell carcinoma.

Q Dysgerminomas:

32 are the most common malignant germ cell tumours

33 are analogous to seminomas in male testes

34 mostly occur in those aged over 30 years

35 comprise 1% of ovarian malignancies

36 are bilateral in 10%–15% of cases

37 secrete hCG in 10%–15% of cases.

Q In endodermal sinus (yolk-sac) tumours:

38 Schiller–Duval body is a histological feature

39 AFP is secreted.

Q Non-gestational choriocarcinoma of the ovary:

40 is a malignant germ cell tumour with a good prognosis

41 responds well to methotrexate or actinomycin D

42 usually develops in women aged 20–30 years.

Q Struma ovarii:

43 is associated with hypothyroidism

44 is usually malignant.

Q Gonadoblastomas:

45 are tumours comprising germ cell and sex cord-stromal elements

46 usually occur in dysgenetic gonads

47 develop in patients with gonadal dysgenesis and a Y chromosome

48 aggressively metastasise, therefore should be removed when suspected.

Q Granulosa-theca cell tumours:

49 histologically feature Call–Exner bodies

50 are associated with delayed puberty

51 typically secrete androgens

52 may secrete oestrogen

53 mostly occur before puberty

54 may cause abnormal uterine bleeding

55 may cause secondary amenorrhoea

56 present in stage I in 90% of cases

57 are usually bilateral tumours

58 have had inhibin, serum oestradiol and serum testosterone used as markers and have been followed serially during treatment.

Q Thecomas:

59 are benign and occur most commonly in young women

60 can be associated with oestrogen production but not as often as in granulosa cell tumours

61 may be associated with hydrothorax and benign ascites.

Q Fibroma of the ovary:

62 is more common in young women

63 often secretes oestrogen

64 may be associated with hydrothorax and benign ascites.

Q Sertoli–Leydig cell tumours:

65 occur mostly in older women

66 are malignant tumours that may cause virilisation

67 have a poor prognosis.

Q With regard to benign breast disease:

68 fibroadenomas change in size during the menstrual cycle

69 severe acute cyclical mastalgia usually responds to treatment with danazol

70 bromocriptine and tamoxifen can be used to treat cyclical mastalgia.

Q With regard to breast carcinoma:
- 71 single-duct discharge from the nipple is strongly associated with carcinoma
- 72 the risk of developing the disease increases with age
- 73 5%–10% of cases have a genetic or familial link
- 74 the BRCA1 gene mutation is present on chromosome 17 and confers a lifetime risk of 50%
- 75 the BRCA2 gene mutation is present on chromosome 13 and confers a lifetime risk of 20%
- 76 the BRCA2 gene mutation is associated with male breast cancer with a 5%–10% lifetime risk
- 77 bilateral oophorectomy before the age of 35 years, without hormonal replacement, reduces risk by 70%
- 78 obese women have a higher risk during post-menopausal years
- 79 the most common breast malignancy is infiltrating ductal carcinoma
- 80 the age at which a woman has her first-term child is more important than parity in estimating risk
- 81 there is increased risk if there is early menarche and late menopause.

Q Each of the following is a sign of breast carcinoma:
- 82 ulceration with signs of inflammation
- 83 induration
- 84 oedema (peau d'orange)
- 85 dimpling
- 86 retraction.

Q With regard to breast cancer:
- 87 bilateral cancer occurs in 10% of cases
- 88 infiltrating lobular carcinoma is more likely than infiltrating ductal carcinoma to involve both breasts
- 89 approximately two-thirds of all women who develop breast cancer eventually develop distant metastases
- 90 the presence and number of axillary node metastases is a predictor of survival.

Q Regarding phyllodes tumours (cystosarcoma phyllodes) of the breast:

   91 they usually present in the fifth decade of life

   92 metastases occur in approximately 10% cases

   93 30% recur within 2–3 years following diagnosis

   94 they metastasise via lymph nodes to the lungs, bone, heart and liver

   95 treatment includes axillary node dissection

   96 most have a poor prognosis.

Q Intraductal papilloma of breast:

   97 classically presents with spontaneous, intermittent blood-stained discharge from both nipples

   98 is most common among perimenopausal women

   99 is associated with increased risk of breast cancer

  100 is treated by excision biopsy.

Q Paget's disease of the breast:

  101 constitutes less than 1% of breast cancers

  102 can appear to resemble eczema or dermatitis of the nipple

  103 has a poor prognosis.

Q With regard to diethylstilbestrol (DES):

  104 it is a potent synthetic oestrogen

  105 DES-exposed female fetuses themselves develop a greater risk of spontaneous miscarriage

  106 a DES-exposed female fetus is more likely to have congenital uterine anomalies

  107 a DES-exposed female fetus is more likely to have a partial transverse vaginal septum

  108 a DES-exposed female fetus is at greater risk of vaginal adenosis

  109 a DES-exposed female fetus will be at increased risk (5%) of having an ectopic pregnancy

  110 a DES-exposed female fetus is at greater risk of squamous cell carcinoma of the vagina.

Q Differential diagnosis of vaginal bleeding in a young person without breast budding typically includes:

111 granulosa cell tumour

112 oestrogen-secreting neoplasia

113 *Shigella flexneri* infection

114 endodermal sinus tumour

115 sarcoma botryoides

116 McCune–Albright syndrome

117 foreign body

118 lichen sclerosis

119 urethral prolapse.

Q With regard to spermicides:

120 nonoxynol 9 is a surfactant

121 nonoxynol 9 destroys the sperm cell membrane

122 a contraceptive sponge, polyurethane impregnated with nonoxynol 9, does not have to be inserted before each act of intercourse, as it remains active for 24 hours once used

123 when used consistently and correctly, the contraceptive sponge is estimated to be approximately 80%–90% effective

124 use of a contraceptive sponge by women who have HIV or acquired immune deficiency syndrome (AIDS) or who are at high risk of HIV is not generally recommended.

Q With regard to barrier methods of contraception:

125 use of the diaphragm is associated with increased rates of UTI

126 the cervical cap should remain in place for at least 2 hours following intercourse, otherwise emergency contraception should be considered

127 women with HIV should not use either the cap or diaphragm

128 both the cervical cap and diaphragm (with spermicide) reduce the risk of sexually transmitted infections

129 the arcing spring diaphragm can be used in women with a retroverted uterus, a rectocele, a cystocele or lax muscle tone.

Q Lactation amenorrhoea as a method of contraception:

130 is over 98% effective

131 requires no long intervals between feeds either during the day or night

132 is effective for less than 9 months post-partum.

Q Examples of UK Medical Eligibility Criteria (UKMEC) category 4 (unacceptable health risk if contraceptive method is used) include:

133 initiating the progestogen-only pill (POP) in women with malignant hepatoma

134 initiating the levonorgestrel (LNG) intrauterine device (IUD) in women with a history of ischaemic heart disease and SLE with antiphospholipid antibodies

135 initiating the combined oral contraceptive pill (COCP) in women who carry the BRCA1 gene mutation.

Q The LNG-IUD (Mirena® intrauterine system [IUS]):

136 has a lower expulsion rate in nulliparous women

137 is relatively contraindicated in women with breast cancer

138 in women with SLE with antiphospholipid antibodies the risks outweigh the benefits of the LNG-IUD (UKMEC category 3)

139 releases 20 mg/24 hours of levonorgestrel.

Q The following are examples of drug interactions:

140 sodium valproate and the COCP

141 topiramate and the COCP

142 phenytoin and depot medroxyprogesterone acetate (DMPA)

143 nucleoside reverse transcriptase inhibitors and the POP

144 non-nucleoside reverse transcriptase inhibitors and progestogen-only implants

145 primidone and the POP

146 lamotrigine and the POP.

Q Enzyme-inducing drugs cause the serum level of ethinylestradiol (EE) to fall such that:

147 30 mg of EE should be taken with sodium valproate

148 50 mg of EE is recommended when taking some antiretroviral treatment for HIV

149 30 mg of EE is recommended when taking rifampicin.

Q   With regard to post-partum contraception:

150   no contraception is required for the first 28 days

151   breastfeeding women should be told that DMPA is not recommended before 6 weeks post-partum

152   troublesome bleeding can occur when DMPA is used less than 6 weeks post-partum

153   in situations where women are at risk of pregnancy and unwilling to consider an alternative, DMPA may be given on day 21 without the need for additional contraceptive cover

154   the cervical cap and diaphragm should not be used before 6 weeks post-partum

155   the COCP must be avoided in breastfeeding.

Q   With regard to progestogen-only injectable injections:

156   they may be used in women up to age of 50 years with regular (2-yearly) reviews

157   they are associated with small loss of bone mineral density, which usually recovers after discontinuation

158   they should not be used in women aged less than 18 years

159   they require that norethisterone enantate (NET-EN) be given intramuscularly every 12 weeks

160   NET-EN is only licensed for short-term use; for example, in women whose partners have undergone vasectomy until vasectomy is proved effective.

Q   With regard to emergency contraception following late administration of progestogen-only injectable injections – that is, 14 weeks + 1 day or longer for DMPA (or 10 weeks + 1 day or longer for NET-EN):

161   within 3 days of unprotected sexual intercourse (UPSI), women may receive emergency contraception or a copper IUD; progestogen-only injectable injection may be given and barrier methods used for 7 days

162   4–5 days after UPSI, women may have a copper IUD inserted; a progestogen-only injectable injection may be given and a pregnancy test should be undertaken 21 days later

163   more than 5 days after UPSI, no emergency contraception should be offered. Barrier methods should be used for 21 days, after which a pregnancy test should be performed; if this pregnancy test is negative, a progestogen-only injectable injection can be given.

Q With regard to women using DMPA:

164 they should have their DMPA injections at 10-weekly intervals when taking enzyme-inducing drugs

165 it can be part of treatment for endometriosis and/or dysmenorrhoea

166 the upper age limit for use is 50 years

167 the average weight gain after 2 years is 8 kg

168 if unacceptable bleeding occurs, in the absence of gynaecological pathology or infection, continuation of DMPA with the addition of mefenamic acid and EE (the combined pill) may be indicated as a short-term measure

169 they should be advised of reduced fertility following cessation

170 they should be told that it works primarily by inhibiting ovulation

171 no maximum duration has been suggested, but women should have 2-yearly reviews and it should be discontinued at age 50.

Q The emergency contraceptive ulipristal acetate (ellaOne®):

172 is thought to work primarily by inhibiting implantation

173 is a selective progesterone receptor modulator

174 one tablet (30 mg) should be taken within 72 hours of UPSI

175 may be used as emergency contraceptive more than once during one menstrual cycle

176 is contraindicated in breastfeeding women

177 is superior to progestogen-only emergency contraception according to pooled data

178 has side effects, which include irregular bleeding, abdominal pain and increased post-treatment cycle length

179 ranitidine, omeprazole and antacids may reduce its efficacy.

Q POPs available in the UK contain:

180 drospirenone

181 desogestrel

182 gestodene

183 ethynodiol diacetate.

Q Women may begin taking the POP if they:

184 suffer from migraine with aura

185 have had breast cancer in the past but no history of the disease for 5 years.

Q If the traditional POP is more than 3 hours late or a desogestrel-only pill is more than 12 hours late, women should be advised to:

186 take the late or missed pill immediately and continue taking the pill at the usual time, even if this means taking two pills together

187 use barrier methods or abstain for the next 7 days.

Q UKMEC 4 (unacceptable health risk if contraceptive method is used) for initiation of the combined contraceptive pill include:

188 secondary Raynaud's disease without lupus anticoagulant

189 smoking 10 cigarettes per day and aged 39 years

Q Features of migraine with aura include:

190 symptoms of aura occur at onset of headache

191 flashing lights

192 scotoma

193 unilateral paraesthesia and/or weakness

194 homonymous hemianopia

195 aphasia or speech defects.

Q Indications for emergency contraception:

196 three 30–35 mcg or two 20 mcg EE pills of the 21 active tablets missed in the third week (pills 14–21)

197 one or more POPs missed or taken more than 3 hours late (more than 12 hours for Cerazette®) and UPSI occurred within 48 hours following the missed tablet(s).

Q With regard to Levonelle 1500®:

198 it cannot be prescribed for a young person under 16 years of age without parental consent

199 it will prevent 84% of expected pregnancies if taken within 72 hours of UPSI

200 women being treated with topiramate should take 3 mg (two tablets) as a single dose as soon as possible within 72 hours of UPSI.

Q Hysteroscopic sterilisation:
201 is supported by NICE guidelines (2009), provided it is subject to clinical governance and audit
202 must be followed by hysterosalpingogram (HSG) in all patients to demonstrate tubal occlusion before other contraceptive measures may be stopped
203 can cause pelvic pain
204 has been shown to have a 90% patient satisfaction rate at 3 months.

Q With regard to the oestradiol valerate/dienogest combined pill (Qlaira®):
205 dienogest has anti-androgenic activity (a third of that of cyproterone acetate)
206 oestradiol valerate is metabolised to oestradiol
207 it has a monophasic dosage regimen
208 it has different missed-pill rules to other combined pills.

Q With regard to Nexplanon®:
209 it is a progestogen-only implant that is bioequivalent to Implanon® and contains 68 mg of etonogestrel
210 it should be inserted 8–10 cm above the medial epicondyle of the humerus
211 the removal technique for Nexplanon® is different to that of Implanon®
212 Nexplanon®, unlike Implanon®, is radiopaque and has a different insertion technique.

Q The contraceptive patch:
213 may be applied to upper outer arm, upper torso (excluding breasts), buttock or lower abdomen
214 should be applied weekly for 4 consecutive weeks
215 if not replaced after 7 days, still has contraceptive protection for a further 2 days.

Q In regard to the combined vaginal ring NuvaRing®:
- 216 it contains latex
- 217 it releases 15 mcg/day of EE and 120 mcg/day of etonogestrel, which avoids first-pass metabolism
- 218 systemic EE exposure is 50% less than that of the 30 mcg EE combined contraceptive pill
- 219 it is inserted weekly for 3 weeks
- 220 it has similar efficacy to the combined contraceptive pill
- 221 it is associated with less breakthrough bleeding and spotting than the combined contraceptive pill
- 222 the most common side effects are headaches, vaginitis and vaginal discharge.

Q With regard to non-hormonal contraception:
- 223 it can be stopped 1 year after the last menstrual period (LMP) in women aged 50 years
- 224 it can be stopped 2 years after the LMP in women aged less than 50 years
- 225 it is accepted practice that a copper IUD (greater than 300 mm^2 Cu) inserted after the age of 40 years can be left in situ until the menopause
- 226 a copper IUD may be left in situ indefinitely in some circumstances.

Q Causes of ambiguous genitalia at birth in infants with 46 XX karyotype include:
- 227 placental aromatase deficiency
- 228 partial gonadal dysgenesis
- 229 CAH
- 230 5-alpha reductase deficiency.

Q Investigations of ambiguous genitalia can include:
- 231 synacthen test
- 232 giving beta-hCG and measuring baseline and post-stimulation levels of androgens
- 233 measuring anti-Müllerian hormone (AMH)
- 234 culture of genital skin.

Q Gonads should be removed before puberty in individuals assigned to female sex with:

235 partial gonadal dysgenesis

236 complete androgen insensitivity syndrome (CAIS)

237 partial androgen insensitivity syndrome

238 dysgenetic gonads.

Q 5-alpha reductase deficiency:

239 is an X-linked condition

240 results in lower conversion of dihydrotestosterone to testosterone

241 can present with ambiguous genitalia

242 is diagnosed by measuring 5-alpha reductase levels in fibroblasts taken from genital skin.

Q Precocious puberty:

243 occurs when the onset of pubertal development starts before the age of 8 years in girls and before 9 years in boys

244 is more common in boys

245 usually occurs in normal sequence

246 is associated with the attainment of shorter adult height

247 that is gonadotrophin dependent accounts for the majority of cases

248 may be caused by central nervous system malformations

249 cases are mostly idiopathic.

Q Gonadotrophin-independent precocious puberty:

250 is found to be the cause in 80% of cases

251 is most commonly caused by an oestrogen-secreting ovarian tumour

252 may be caused by choriocarcinoma.

Q McCune–Albright syndrome may be:

253 associated with café au lait spots

254 associated with polyostotic dysplasia

255 associated with cysts of skull and long bones

256 associated with facial asymmetry

257 associated with gonadotrophin-dependent puberty

258 treated with aromatase inhibitors.

Q Treatment of precocious puberty with gonadotrophin-releasing hormone (GnRH) analogues has been shown to:

259 cause regression of breast development and pubic hair

260 decrease growth velocity by around 50%

261 render all girls amenorrhoeic

262 return sex steroid hormones to prepubertal range within 2 weeks

263 restore normal height with the addition of growth hormone.

Q Delayed puberty:

264 is defined as the absence of all secondary sexual characteristics by the age of 16 years

265 may result from excessive exercise

266 is associated with galactosaemia

267 is associated with diabetes mellitus

268 is associated with pituitary adenoma

269 is associated with Swyer syndrome

270 is associated with Kallman's syndrome.

Q Management of delayed puberty:

271 involves the induction of puberty using high-dose EE

272 caused by hypergonadotrophic hypogonadism includes the use of pulsatile gonadotrophins given subcutaneously.

Q Primary amenorrhoea may be caused by:

273 mumps

274 kernicterus

275 hypothyroidism

276 thalassaemia major

277 retinitis pigmentosa.

Q Deficiency in 17 alpha-hydroxylase with 46 XX karyotype is associated with:

278 virilisation

279 hyponatraemia

280 hyperkalaemia

281 hypogonadism

282 secondary amenorrhoea.

Q Recognised causes of secondary amenorrhoea include:

283 levodopa

284 empty sella syndrome

285 lymphocytic hypophysitis

286 sarcoidosis

287 pseudocyesis

288 excessive exercise

289 late-onset CAH

290 diabetes mellitus

291 Cushing's disease.

Q Premature ovarian failure may be associated with:

292 Cushing's disease

293 Hashimoto's thyroiditis

294 hypoparathyroidism.

Q With regard to premature ovarian failure:

295 karyotyping should be performed in all cases

296 gonads should be biopsied at laparoscopy

297 clomiphene may be used to induce ovulation.

Q Primary dysmenorrhoea:

298 occurs in 75% of young women

299 is more common in smokers

300 is less likely to occur in women who have had children born vaginally

301 is associated with increased prostaglandin F2alpha.

Q Recognised causes of primary dysmenorrhoea include:

302 stress

303 conditioned behaviour

304 congenital obstructed Müllerian malformations.

Q Recognised causes of dysmenorrhoea include:

305 cervical stenosis

306 endometriosis

307 adenomyosis

308 uterine polyp.

Q Somatic symptoms of premenstrual syndrome may include:

309 thirst

310 change in bowel habit

311 breast pain

312 poor coordination

313 hot flushes.

Q Affective symptoms of premenstrual syndrome may include:

314 subjective confusion

315 lethargy

316 insomnia

317 social withdrawal

318 paranoid thoughts

319 auditory hallucinations

320 depression

321 anxiety

322 flight of ideas

323 mood lability

324 impulsivity.

Q Premenstrual syndrome:

325 has a lower prevalence among Hispanics

326 is more prevalent among those with higher education

327 is less prevalent among smokers.

Q Lichen sclerosis is associated with:

328 squamous hyperplasia

Q Lichen sclerosis:

329 appears hyperkeratotic

330 affects limbs and the trunk.

Q Treatment options for vulval intraepithelial neoplasia include:

331 imiquimod

332 simple vulvectomy.

Q Treatment of vaginal intraepithelial neoplasia (VAIN) 3 typically involves:

333 laser vaporisation

334 vaginectomy.

Q Known risk factors for developing vulval carcinoma include:

335 lichen planus

336 Paget's disease

337 human papillomavirus (HPV) serotypes 31 and 33

338 HPV serotypes 6 and 11.

Q With regard to male factor infertility:

339 hyperprolactinaemia causes impotence

340 hyperprolactinaemia causes oligospermia

341 varicoceles are associated with infertility and conception rates improve after surgical correction

342 varicoceles are more common on the right

343 microdeletions on the Y chromosome are associated with azoospermia

344 microdeletions on the Y chromosome are associated with oligospermia.

Q Anovulatory infertility:

345 is the most common cause of female infertility

346 caused by polycystic ovary syndrome (PCOS) is typically hypergonadotrophic.

Q Infertility resulting from tubal damage may be caused by:

347 Crohn's disease

348 septic miscarriage

349 endometriosis.

Q With regard to tubal disease:

350 proximal disease accounts for 75% of cases

351 microsurgical reconstruction is successful in 50%–60% of cases

352 bilateral salpingectomies for hydrosalpinges improve IVF success rates.

Q Risk factors for developing ovarian hyperstimulation syndrome (OHSS) include:

353 age over 35 years

354 obesity

355 hCG administration

356 rapidly rising oestradiol

357 multiple pregnancy.

Q Prevention of OHSS includes:

358 withholding hCG

359 luteal support using progesterone rather than hCG

360 withholding embryo transfer.

Q Recurrent miscarriage:

361 affects 5% of women

362 is caused by abnormal parental karyotype, the most common of which is a Robertsonian translocation

363 may be caused by antithrombin III deficiency

364 may be caused by a subseptate uterus

365 may be caused by elevated proteins C and S.

Q Ectopic pregnancies are more common in:

366 chromosomally abnormal conceptions

367 older women

368 women who smoke

369 the isthmic rather than the ampullary portion of the tube.

Q Risk factors for gestational trophoblastic disease include:

370 diets deficient in folic acid, vitamin A and protein

371 women with blood group A whose partners have blood group O

372 women with AB blood group

373 maternal age less than 16 or greater than 40 years.

Q Complete moles:

374 are diploid

375 result from androgenesis

376 are typically formed by dispermy.

Q Incomplete moles:

377 are triploid

378 can occur with a phenotypically normal fetus

379 comprise hyperplastic syncytiotrophoblasts.

Q Placental-site trophoblastic tumours:

380 secrete human placental lactogen, which may be used as a tumour marker

381 metastases develop in 50% of cases

382 are treated by hysterectomy

383 respond well to treatment with methotrexate.

Q Features of hydatidiform mole:

384 presents with abnormal bleeding

385 uterus small for dates

386 theca-lutein cysts

387 pre-eclampsia

388 hypothyroidism

389 may present with ovarian torsion

390 may result in pulmonary oedema

391 may result in disseminated intravascular coagulopathy

392 are more common in South East Asia

393 complete moles are more common than partial moles.

Q With regard to hyperandrogenism:

394 the free androgen index (FAI) is a measure of active testosterone that relies on measurement of both free testosterone and sex hormone-binding protein (SHBG)

395 virilisation is usually associated with markedly elevated levels of testosterone

396 hypertrichosis is a feature of virilisation

397 virilisation is associated with temporal balding

398 the major androgen produced by the ovary is testosterone

399 the major androgen produced by the adrenal gland is dehydroepiandrosterone (DHEA)

400 stromal hyperthecosis is associated with bilaterally enlarged ovaries and elevated levels of testosterone.

Q With regard to PCOS:

401 15%–20% of women with PCOS have mildly elevated prolactin

402 most women of normal BMI with PCOS have insulin resistance

403 acanthosis nigricans is associated with PCOS

404 it is associated with elevated homocysteine, endothelin-1 and reduced plasminogen activator inhibitor-1

405 women with PCOS are at increased risk of death due to ischaemic heart disease.

Q Excess androgen in pregnancy can be caused by:

406 luteoma

407 hyperreactio luteinalis

408 benign mature teratoma.

Q Dermoid cysts have been known to cause:

409 hyperthyroidism

410 carcinoid syndrome

411 autoimmune haemolytic anaemia

412 more commonly, rupture in pregnancy.

Q The menopause occurs earlier in:

413 smokers

414 Down's syndrome

415 women with high parity

416 the indigenous population of Malay.

Q Recognised symptoms associated with the menopause include:

417 dyspareunia

418 vulval itching

419 urinary frequency and dysuria

420 long-term memory loss

421 night sweats.

Q Effective treatments for vasomotor symptoms in menopausal women include:

422 red clover

423 St John's wort

424 acupuncture

425 phytoestrogens

426 clonidine

427 venlafaxine.

Q Risks and benefits of hormone replacement therapy (HRT) include:

428 apparent significant reduction in the risk of colorectal cancer for duration of HRT treatment

429 increased risk of dementia in women older than 65 years

430 increased risk of gallbladder disease

431 decreased risk of myocardial infarction.

Q Diagnosis of bacterial vaginosis requires:

432 absence of lactobacilli

433 presence of clue cells

434 pH < 4.5.

Q *Trichomonas* vaginal infection:

435 is highly infectious and sexually transmitted

436 causes cervicitis, 'strawberry cervix', in 30% of cases

437 is caused by a unicellular, aerobic flagellated protozoan

438 is associated with a frothy malodorous discharge in 25% of cases.

Q Candidiasis ('thrush'):

439 is caused by a Gram-positive fungi

440 is predominantly an infection during childbearing years

441 is more common in obese women

442 is associated with a pH > 6

443 may cause fissuring

444 may be diagnosed following culture in Sabouraud medium.

Q With regard to genital tract infection:

445 *Trichomonas vaginalis* resides in Skene's glands and lower urinary tract as well as vagina

446 condyloma acuminatum is the most common sexually transmitted disease in the UK

447 *Molluscum contagiosum* is usually a self-limiting infection

448 *Haemophilus ducreyi* is a Gram-negative rod that causes a painless chancre

449 lymphogranuloma venereum is a chronic infection caused by *Chlamydia trachomatis* and is associated with Donovan bodies.

Q With regard to syphilis:

450 it is caused by an anaerobic spirochaete with an incubation period of 14 days

451 patients remain contagious during both primary and secondary syphilis

452 the Venereal Disease Research Laboratory (VDRL) test is a specific test for *Treponema pallidum*

453 EIA, FTA and TPHA are specific tests for *T. pallidum* and, following infection, remain positive for life

454 it is associated with the Jarisch–Herxheimer reaction following treatment

455 fetal infection can cause polyhydramnios and hydrops fetalis.

Q Toxic shock syndrome is associated with:

456 *Staphylococcus aureus* infection and endotoxin TSST-1

457 desquamation of skin

458 rashes that may resemble severe sunburn.

Q With regard to *Neisseria gonorrhoeae* infection:

459 nucleic acid amplification testing of urine or cervix is the most sensitive diagnostic test

460 the majority of women who have gonorrhoea are asymptomatic

461 haematogenous spread to joints can occur

462 it is caused by a Gram-negative rod.

Q Fitz-Hugh–Curtis syndrome:

463 is a recognised cause of pleuritic pain

464 is a recognised cause of shoulder tip pain

465 may be caused by coxsackievirus.

Q With regard to pelvic tuberculosis:

466 it is caused by both *Mycobacterium tuberculosis* and *Mycobacterium bovis*

467 the primary site of infection is usually the lung

468 it causes abnormal uterine bleeding

469 the predominant site of infection is the uterus.

Q With regard to hepatitis B:

470 investigations characteristically demonstrate presence of anti-HBs in acute infection

471 investigations characteristically demonstrate elevated HBeAg in chronic high infectivity

472 chronic high infectivity typically has a presence of hepatitis B virus DNA and HBsAg.

Q Complications of posterior colporrhaphy include:

473 pudendal neuralgia

474 worsening of bowel symptoms

475 injury to the genitofemoral nerve

476 dyspareunia, which is less likely to occur if surgical placation of levator ani is performed.

Q With regard to pelvic posterior compartment prolapse:

477 a proctogram is recommended if obstructed defecation is suspected

478 a stapled transanal rectal resection is designed to treat rectal intussusception.

Q Urinary incontinence is associated with:

479 obesity

480 pregnancy

481 hysterectomy in older women

482 dementia.

Q Overactive bladder syndrome is:

483 urgency, frequency and nocturia without urge urinary incontinence.

Q Video cystourethrography:

484 involves the use of contrast medium to fill the bladder

485 is useful when neurological causes for urinary dysfunction are suspected

486 can demonstrate reflux.

Q There is good evidence for the treatment of urge urinary incontinence using:

487 trospium chloride

488 propiverine

489 amitriptyline.

Q Liquid-based cytology for cervical screening has the following advantages over conventional smear test:

490 it is more sensitive

491 it can test for HPV and *C. trachomatis*

492 it reduces the number of inadequate smears.

Q According to FIGO staging (2009) for carcinoma of the vulva:

493 Stage IB: the tumour is confined to the vulva or perineum; is greater than 2 cm or, with stromal invasion, is greater than 1 mm; and has negative nodes

494 Stage II: the tumour is of any size with adjacent spread (one-third of the lower urethra, one-third of the lower vagina, anus) and negative nodes

495 Stage IIIA: the tumour is of any size with positive inguino-femoral lymph nodes

496 Stage IIIB: two or more lymph nodes metastases greater than or equal to 5 mm

497 Stage IIIC: the node or nodes are positive with extracapsular spread

498 Stage IVA (i): the tumour invades other regional structures (two-thirds of the upper urethra, two-thirds of the upper vagina) and bladder mucosa and/or rectal mucosa, or is fixed to the pelvic bone

499 Stage IVA (ii): fixed or ulcerated inguino-femoral lymph nodes

500 Stage IVB: any distant metastasis including pelvic lymph nodes.

Q According to FIGO staging (2009) for carcinoma of the endometrium:

501 Stage IA: the tumour is confined to the uterus with none or less than half of the myometrium invaded

502 Stage IB: the tumour is confined to the uterus, with more than half of the myometrium invaded.

Q According to FIGO staging (2009) for uterine sarcomas (leiomyosarcoma, endometrial stromal sarcoma and adenosarcoma):

503 Stage IA: the tumour is limited to the uterus and is less than 5 cm

504 Stage IB: the tumour is limited to the uterus and is greater than 5 cm

505 Stage IIA: the tumour extends to the pelvis and there is adnexal involvement

506 Stage IIB: the tumour extends to extra-uterine pelvic tissue

507 Stage IIIA: the tumour invades abdominal tissues, one site

508 Stage IIIB: there is more than one site

509 Stage IIIC: there is metastasis to pelvic and/or para-aortic lymph nodes

510 Stage IVA: the tumour invades the bladder and/or rectum

511 Stage IVB: there is distant metastasis.

Q Common side effects of the HPV vaccine include:

512 vomiting

513 itchy skin

514 red skin rash

515 joint pain

516 pyrexia of greater than 38°C.

Q HPV vaccination:

517 consists of three doses and all three injections are needed to ensure full protection against the virus

518 is given in secondary schools to girls aged 12–13 years.

Q Cervarix® (the HPV vaccine used in the UK vaccination programme):

519 protects against HPV-16

520 protects against HPV-18

521 guarantees to prevent cervical cancer

522 protects against genital warts.

Q   With regard to uterine sarcomas:

523   radiotherapy has been shown to reduce the risk of local recurrence

524   they commonly metastasise to lungs

525   the risk of developing uterine sarcoma is increased 5–25 years following pelvic radiotherapy.

Q   Carcinoma of the fallopian tube:

526   is usually unilateral

527   is more common in perimenopausal women

528   more commonly has metastatic causes

529   is usually adenocarcinoma

530   has elevated CA125 in the majority of cases.

Q   With regard to ovarian carcinoma:

531   it is the most common gynaecological malignancy in the UK

532   breast cancer is the most common primary site for metastatic ovarian tumour

533   use of the COCP increases the risk.

Q   In the presence of pregnancy of unknown location, serum progesterone levels:

534   less than 20 nmol/L predict spontaneous pregnancy resolution

535   more than 60 nmol/L are strongly associated with pregnancies subsequently shown to be normal.

Q   Prior to surgical uterine evacuation:

536   routine antibiotic prophylaxis is recommended.

Q   The following symptoms are associated with endometriosis:

537   dysmenorrhoea

538   superficial dyspareunia

539   subfertility

540   chronic fatigue

541   dyschezia.

Q Recommendations for management of endometriosis include:

542 laparoscopic ovarian cystectomy for endometriomas greater than 5 cm in diameter.

543 treatment with a GnRH antagonist for 3–6 months before IVF in women with endometriosis increases the rate of clinical pregnancy.

Q Regarding gestational trophoblastic disease:

544 the incidence in the UK is 1/1600 live births

545 there is higher incidence in women in the Afro-Caribbean population

546 incidence after a live birth is estimated at 1/100 000

547 10% of partial moles represent tetraploid or mosaic conceptions

548 there is usually evidence of a fetus or fetal red blood cell in partial mole

549 the risk of future molar pregnancy is 1/1000.

Q Regarding follow-up of gestational trophoblastic disease:

550 if hCG levels have reverted to normal within 56 days of the pregnancy event, then follow-up will be for 6 months from the date of uterine evacuation

551 if hCG levels have not reverted to normal within 56 days of the pregnancy event, then follow-up will be for 6 months from normalisation of these levels

552 intrauterine contraceptive devices should not be used until hCG levels are normal to reduce the risk of gestational trophoblastic neoplasia

553 single-agent progestogens are preferable to the COCP once hCG levels are normal.

Q Chemotherapy is needed following diagnosis of:

554 complete mole in 15% of cases

555 partial mole in 0.5% of cases.

Q In VTE:

556 the incidence in post-menopausal women is four times more than that of premenopausal women

557 myeloproliferative disorders are a recognised risk factor.

Q The incidence of complications associated with laparoscopic procedures:
  558 intestinal injuries: 0.6/1000
  559 urological injuries: 0.3/1000
  560 vascular injuries: 0.1/1000.

Q The rate of adhesion formation at umbilicus following abdominal surgery:
  561 is 80% with midline laparotomy
  562 is 40% with low transverse incision.

Q After an IVF cycle, the incidence of:
  563 mild OHSS is 33%
  564 moderate or severe OHSS is 3%–8%.

Q Diagnosis of OHSS may include:
  565 abdominal bloating
  566 vomiting
  567 oliguria
  568 haematocrit less than 45%
  569 hyperproteinaemia
  570 hydrothorax
  571 leukocytosis.

Q Complications of pregnancies associated with OHSS include:
  572 thromboembolism
  573 miscarriage
  574 pregnancy-induced hypertension
  575 premature delivery.

Q PCOS is associated with
  576 endometrial hyperplasia
  577 breast cancer
  578 ovarian cancer
  579 type 1 diabetes
  580 hypertension.

Q In comparison with rigid hysteroscopy, with outpatient flexible hysteroscopy:

581 there is less pain

582 images are better

583 there are fewer failed procedures

584 examination is quicker

585 costs are reduced.

Q In outpatient diagnostic hysteroscopy:

586 a chaperone is needed only for male clinicians

587 instillation of local anaesthetic into the cervical canal does not reduce pain during the procedure

588 instillation of local anaesthetic into the cervical canal may reduce the incidence of vasovagal reactions

589 vaginoscopy reduces pain during diagnostic rigid outpatient hysteroscopy.

Q Long-term complications of colposuspension include:

590 voiding difficulty in 20% of cases

591 de novo detrusor overactivity in 40% of cases

592 genitourinary prolapse in 13% of cases.

Q Sling procedures, using autologous or synthetic materials, may result in:

593 a continence rate of 50%

594 a risk of vaginal erosion of up to 36%

595 a risk of urethral erosion of up to 15%

596 de novo detrusor overactivity of up to 66%

597 in up to 35% of cases, procedures requiring sling revision or removal

598 10% risk of some voiding disorder symptoms subsequent to the immediate post-operative period

599 9% risk of long-term self-catheterisation.

Q Complications of sacrocolpopexy include:

600 bladder injury

601 incisional hernia

602 mesh rejection

603 rectovaginal haematoma

604 vaginal pain.

Q Medical conditions that increase the risk of VTE include:

605 varicose veins

606 superficial thrombophlebitis.

Q Lifetime risk of developing invasive vulval cancer with

607 lichen sclerosis 2%–4%

608 lichen planus 2%–4%.

Q Complications from abdominal hysterectomy include:

609 bladder injury in 7/1000

610 ureteric injury in 7/1000

611 bowel injury in 7/1000

612 haemorrhage requiring blood transfusion in 50/1000

613 return to theatre in 7/1000

614 pelvic infection in 7/1000

615 VTE in 4/1000.

Q Complications from diagnostic hysteroscopy include:

616 infertility

617 failure to complete intended procedure.

Q Laparoscopy for gynaecological indications:

618 may result in death in 3–8/100 000

619 may result in persistent trophoblastic tissue when salpingostomy is performed for ectopic pregnancy in 20/100

620 has a lifetime failure rate of 5/1000 for laparoscopic tubal occlusion.

Q The risks of surgical evacuation of retained products include:

621 uterine perforation 5/1000

622 infertility

623 blood transfusion 5/1000

624 need for repeat surgical evacuation 5/1000

625 pelvic infection 10/1000.

Q Complications associated with vaginal surgery for prolapse include:

626 bladder injury in 2/1000

627 bowel injury in 5/1000

628 pelvic abscess in 3/1000

629 death within 6 weeks in 37/100 000.

Q Regarding fertility:

630 84% of couples in the general population will conceive within 1 year if they do not use contraception and have regular sexual intercourse

631 92% of couples in the general population will conceive within 2 years if they do not use contraception and have regular sexual intercourse

632 94% of fertile women aged 35 years will conceive after 3 years of trying

633 77% of those aged 38 years will conceive after 3 years of trying.

Q The World Health Organization (2010) reference values for semen analysis are as follows:

634 volume: 1.5 mL or more

635 total sperm number: more than 39 million/ejaculate

636 sperm concentration: 15 million spermatozoa per mL

637 motility: 40% or more motile (grades A and B)

638 vitality: greater than 58% viable

639 white blood cells: fewer than 1 million per mL

640 morphology: 4% strictly normal

641 any morphological defects: less than 20%.

Q The chances of a live birth per treatment cycle of assisted reproduction treatment (IVF) are:

642 greater than 20% for women aged 23–35 years

643 15% for women aged 36–38 years

644 10% for women aged 39 years

645 6% for women aged 40 years or older.

Q The following interventions during IVF cycles improve pregnancy rates:

646 the use of adjuvant growth hormone with gonadotrophins

647 assisted hatching

648 blastocyst transfer

649 ultrasound-guided embryo transfer

650 embryo transfers on day 2 or 3 rather than on day 5 or 6

651 embryo transfer into a uterine cavity with an endometrium thickness of less than 5 mm

652 bed rest of greater than 20 minutes' duration following embryo transfer.

Q Complications of uterine artery embolisation (UAE) include:

653 persistent vaginal discharge

654 vomiting

655 premature ovarian failure

656 haematoma.

Q With regard to endometrial ablation for the management of menorrhagia:

657 it may be offered as an initial treatment

658 it can be offered with uterine fibroids of up to 5 cm in diameter.

659 uterine size up to 12 weeks

660 second-generation ablation techniques should be used as first-line treatment

661 transcervical resection of the endometrium is appropriate if hysteroscopic myomectomy is included in the procedure.

Q Risks associated with IUDs include:

662 uterine perforation at the time of IUD insertion in 1/1000

663 pelvic inflammatory disease following IUD insertion in 1/100

664 expulsion of IUD within 5 years in 1/100

665 overall risk of ectopic pregnancy within 5 years in 1/100

666 ectopic pregnancy in 1/100 if the woman becomes pregnant with the IUD in situ.

Q Risks associated with the Mirena® coil include:

667 uterine perforation at the time of IUD insertion in 1/1000

668 pelvic inflammatory disease following IUD insertion in 1/100

669 expulsion of IUD within 5 years in 1/100

670 overall risk of ectopic pregnancy within 5 years in 1/100

671 the risk of ectopic pregnancy in 1/100 if the woman becomes pregnant with the IUD in situ.

Q The IUS:

672 is contraindicated for use in nulliparous women

673 can be used safely by breastfeeding women

674 is not contraindicated for use in women with diabetes

675 is contraindicated for use in women who are HIV positive or have AIDS

676 can be fitted from 6 weeks post-partum, irrespective of the mode of delivery.

Q Newer treatment modalities of fibroids include:

677 magnetic resonance (MR) image-guided percutaneous laser ablation

678 MR image-guided transcutaneous focused ultrasound ablation

679 iliac artery embolisation.

3
Statistics

Q Normal distribution possesses the following important mathematical properties:
1 it is always symmetrical
2 the mean, median and mode all have the same value
3 no matter how far the tails of the curve are followed, they never reach the horizontal axis
4 if the mean and standard deviation (SD) of a normal distribution are known, the normal distribution curve can be drawn.

Q Regarding the SD of a normally distributed set of data:
5 34% of the data scores fall within one SD above the mean
6 99.73% of the population is accounted for by two SD above and below the mean
7 to calculate the SD, the standard (z) scores are required.

Q The two graphical techniques of histograms and bar charts are very similar, but:
8 bar charts are typically used to present interval/ratio data
9 histograms are typically used to present nominal and ordinal data.

Q In the series 3 7 10 19 22 25 25 25, the median is:
10 25
11 $\dfrac{19 + 22}{2}$

Q A trainee conducted a study of how far each woman was able to walk (podometry) in the first 48 hours following an elective caesarean section. She set this data against the woman's BMI, which was measured preoperatively. Having plotted the scatter graph shown (Figure 1), she ran the Pearson test to establish whether there was a significant correlation. The Pearson test shows that the data have a P value of less than 0.005. From this, it can be deduced:
12 there is a statistically significant positive correlation between BMI and distance walked following caesarean section in this cohort
13 as the P value is less than 0.005, there is a significant causal relationship between obesity and reduced mobility following caesarean section
14 the Pearson test is a non-parametric test

15 the Pearson test may be used for correlational designs that compare two sets of data for their degree of association and may be used on ordinal data.

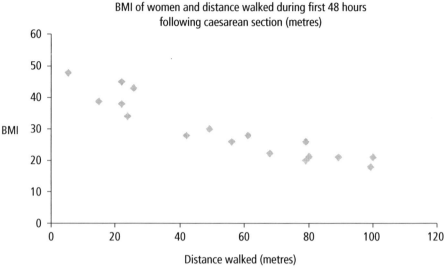

BMI of women and distance walked during first 48 hours following caesarean section (metres)

FIGURE 1 Scatter graph.

Q Regarding Type I errors:

16 they occur when the experimental hypothesis has been supported statistically but when the null (no relationship) hypothesis is, in fact, true

17 they may be avoided by ensuring the selected significance level is appropriate

18 the chance of making a Type I error can be avoided by increasing the sample size

19 replication of the study and its findings reduces the chance of Type I errors

20 can be reduced by using a less-stringent significance level.

Q Type II errors:

21 occur when the experimental hypothesis is rejected in favour of the null (no relationship) hypothesis when the experimental hypothesis is, in fact, true

22 can be safeguarded against using a less-stringent significance level

23 can be safeguarded against by increasing sample size.

Q The chi-square (χ^2) test:

24 may be used when the experimental data uses two matched groups that are compared on, for example, an outcome, task or activity

25 requires the data to be nominal

26 is an example of a parametric test.

Q A trainee hypothesised that women given preoperative counselling 48 hours prior to undergoing caesarean section differ in their levels of post-operative anxiety (measured by a questionnaire scoring on a scale from 0 to 6) according to whether counselling is provided by either specialist midwives or consultant psychiatrists.

27 This is an example of a two-tailed hypothesis.

28 Had the hypothesis predicted that midwives would have greater success than psychiatrists in reducing post-operative anxiety, it would have been a one-tailed hypothesis.

29 In a two-tailed hypothesis, there is twice the possibility of random error accounting for the results.

30 The Mann–Whitney test may be used in this scenario.

31 Unpaired t test may be used in this scenario.

Q Regarding Table 1 concerning a screening test:

32 the sensitivity of the test is calculated by dividing the true positives (a) by the total number of persons affected by the disease (a + c)

33 specificity is calculated by dividing the true negatives (d) by the total number of persons not affected by the disease (b + d)

34 as the sensitivity of a screening test increases, the number of false positives will decrease

35 as the specificity of a screening test increases, the number of false negatives will decrease.

TABLE 1

Screening test result	True status – disease present	True status – disease not present
Positive	a	b
Negative	c	d

Q The predictive value of a screening test is determined by:

36 the sensitivity and specificity of the test

37 the prevalence of the condition that is being tested.

Answers
Obstetrics

1 **F** – damage to dividing cells that may lead to cancer later in life is thought to be proportional to the dose of radiation but can occur at any dose.

2 **T** – radiation damage causing loss of organ function, malformation and death is thought to have a threshold greater than 100 mGy.

3 **T**

4 **T***

5 **T***

6 **T***

*UDP is characteristically associated with abnormal growth patterns and rates of growth. There is no consistent cytogenetic abnormality. It occurs when one homologous chromosome pair comes from the same parent.

7 **T**

8 **F** – dominant inheritance.

9 **F** – X-linked.

10 **F** – X-linked.

11 **T**

12 **T**

13 **T**

14 **T**

15 **F** – dominant.

16 **F** – dominant.

17 **T**

18 **F** – X-linked.

19 **T**

20 **T**

21 **F**

22 **F** – 10%.

23 **F** – 1% – gamete selection is thought to reduce risk further.

24 **F** – 47 XXY.

25 **T** – investigation for fertility.

26 **F** – infertility (azoospermia) is usual except in mosaics.

27 **T** – small increased risk.

28 **F** – recurrence does not appear to be above general population risk – 1:1000 males.

29 **T**

30 **T** – hypocalcaemia is the cause of neonatal seizures.

31 **T**

32 **F** – hypotelorism due to holoprosencephaly.

33   T
34   T
35   T – 8%.
36   T
37   T – 1%–5%.
38   F – increased MCHC.
39   T
40   T
41   T
42   T
43   F – seen in Duchenne and Becker muscular dystrophies.
44   T
45   T
46   T
47   T
48   T – 1%.
49   T
50   F – short stature (70% of normal height) is sometimes called 'male Turner syndrome'.
51   T
52   T
53   T
54   T
55   T
56   T
57   T
58   T
59   T
60   T
61   F – sagittal view.
62   T
63   T
64   T
65   F – 95% transabdominal.
66   F – maximal subcutaneous thickness between fetal skin and soft tissue overlying cervical spine.
67   T
68   F

69 **F**

70 **T**

71 **T** – all reduced apart from hCG and inhibin A.

72 **T** – combined test.

73 **T** – serum integrated test.

74 **F** – PAPP-A is measured between 11 and 13 weeks of gestation. The median value is approximately 0.5 multiples of the median (MoM). Low PAPP-A is associated with trisomy 21, IUGR and pre-eclampsia. The significance of raised PAPP-A is uncertain.

75 **F** – the quadruple test does not meet the standard and should be used only for late booker.

76 **F** – eurofetus data.

77 **F** – case series have reported 60%–70%.

78 **T** – at 20 weeks.

79 **T**

80 **T** – numbers were small. Doppler recordings should not be used in low-risk populations, as false-positive findings can lead to unnecessary iatrogenic preterm delivery.

81 **T** – the umbilical artery Doppler index correlates with placental dysfunction more reliably between 24 and 33 weeks of gestation.

82 **T** – placental resistance decreases with gestation. The umbilical artery Doppler index reflects placental blood flow resistance (determined by architecture of villous vascular tree). As gestation advances, resistance decreases; therefore, umbilical artery Dopplers should not be used in isolation in suspected IUGR (greater than or equal to 34/40) caused by placental dysfunction – instead, middle cerebral artery (MCA) Dopplers should be used. Conventionally, M1 (first segment) should be used, as M2 is always higher. Redistribution of blood is indicated by low middle cerebral artery PI or RI but no randomised controlled trials are available. IVC and ductus venosus Doppler indices, together with umbilical vein pulsations, correctly predict acidaemia in a significant number of cases of IUGR. However, they are technically difficult and cannot be measured in all cases.

83 **T**

84 **T**

85 **T**

86 **T**

87 **T**

88   **T**

89   **T**

90   **F** – male.

91   **T**

92   **T**

93   **T**

94   **F**

95   **T**

96   **T** – any structural anomaly that dilates atria.

97   **T** – in 30%–40% of cases.

98   **F** – rarely responds; sotalol is required.

99   **T**

100   **T**

101   **T**

102   **T** – SLE, Sjögren's syndrome and rheumatoid arthritis are all associated with increased risk of CCHB.

103   **F** – 1%–2%.

104   **T**

105   **T** – pre-pregnancy genetic screening may be offered if maternal tetralogy of Fallot.

106   **F** – aplasia or hypoplasia of thymus with concomitant immunological deficiency.

107   **T**

108   **T**

109   **T**

110   **T**

111   **T**

112   **T**

113   **F** – there is greater incidence in males than in females.

114   **T**

115   **T**

116   **T**

117   **T**

118   **F** – oligohydramnios.

119   **F** – oligohydramnios.

120   **T**

121   **T** – rare.

122   **T** – 'mirror' syndrome.

123 **F** – used in second and early third trimester. There is risk of ductal closure if used later in the third trimester.

124 **T**

125 **T**

126 **T**

127 **T**

128 **F** – 10%.

129 **T**

130 **T**

131 **T**

132 **T**

133 **T**

134 **T**

135 **T** – dolichocephaly can distort findings.

136 **T**

137 **F** – prognosis is highly variable.

138 **T**

139 **T**

140 **T**

141 **T**

142 **T**

143 **T**

144 **T**

145 **F**

146 **F** – more common. Chromosomal abnormality more likely in this situation.

147 **F**

148 **F** – right.

149 **T** – serial growth scans are indicated.

150 **T**

151 **T**

152 **T**

153 **T** – digital hypoplasia and dysmorphic facies.

154 **T**

155 **T**

156 **T**

157 **F** – 60%. Right-sided hernia is technically very difficult to detect.

158 **T** – right-sided has a worse prognosis.

159 **T** – impaired swallowing.

160 **T** – VACTER: Vertebral, Anorectal, Cardiac, Tracheal, oEsophageal, Radial and Renal.

161 **T**

162 **F** – duodenal atresia.

163 **T** – triploidy/trisomy 18.

164 **T** – rarely; the majority are sporadic.

165 **T**

166 **T**

167 **T** – autosomal recessive inheritance.

168 **F** – isolated cases have very good prognosis.

169 **T** – 25% recurrence only in apple peel syndrome (autosomal recessive disorder). The majority have a low risk of recurrence.

170 **F** – 2%–14%.

171 **T**

172 **T**

173 **T**

174 **T**

175 **T**

176 **T**

177 **T**

178 **T**

179 **T** – this is a sign of bowel perforation.

180 **F** – 85% are unilateral.

181 **F** – from pulmonary circulation. The differential diagnosis is bronchopulmonary sequestration, which derives its supply from the aorta.

182 **T**

183 **T**

184 **T**

185 **F** – 5 females:1 male.

186 **T**

187 **T** – they originate from midline structures.

188 **T**

189 **T**

190 **F** – at 1–3 weeks. Assessment that is too early results in higher false negatives.

191 **F** – males.

192 **T**

193 **T**

194 **F** – males.

195 **T**

196 **T**

197 **F** – equinovarus – sole medially.

198 **T**

199 **F** – only if other markers.

200 **F**

201 **F**

202 **T** – uncommon.

203 **T** – transplacental passage of TSH receptor-stimulating antibodies.

204 **T**

205 **F** – 'banana' and 'lemon' signs.

206 **T** – also 'champagne bottle cork'.

207 **T**

208 **T**

209 **T**

210 **T**

211 **F** – 50%.

212 **F** – teratogenic in rodents but not in humans.

213 **T**

214 **T**

215 **F** – less than 1%.

216 **F** – less than 1%.

217 **T** – therefore, follow-up scans are required.

218 **T**

219 **T**

220 **F** – it is a DNA virus of the Herpesviridae family.

221 **T**

222 **F** – infection is more likely in the third trimester.

223 **T**

224 **F** – optic atrophy.

225 **T**

226 **T**

227 **T**

228 **T**

229 **T**

230 **F**

231 **F** – 10%, i.e. 4/40.

232 **T**

233 **T**

234 **T**

235 **T**

236 **F**

238 **T**

239 **T**

240 **T**

241 **F** – Gram positive.

242 **T**

243 **F** – diagnosed by culture of blood, placenta, etc.

244 **T**

245 **F** – ampicillin/gentamicin/erythromycin. It tends to be resistant to cephalosporins.

246 **T**

247 **T**

248 **T**

249 **T**

250 **T**

251 **T**

252 **T**

253 **F** – the Sabin-Feldman dye test is used to measure IgG. Remember IgM alone is unreliable as it can persist for years after infection and therefore its measurement results in many false positives. Toxoplasmosis is diagnosed when IgG shows a ×4 increase over 3 weeks. Can be diagnosed IgM positive and IgG negative but not in all cases; therefore, serial tests should be employed.

254 **T**

255 **T**

256 **T**

257 **F** – lower transmission but greater risk of serious sequelae.

258 **T** – 15% in first trimester.

259 **T**

260 **T** – ventricular dilatation.

261 **T**

262 **T**

263 **T**

264 **F**

265 **F** – greatest risk in puerperium (x20); 2–3× risk in pregnancy.

266 **F** – most are due to arteriovenous malformation (AVM) in pregnancy, as AVM is oestrogen-sensitive. The ratio of berry aneurysm to AVM is 7:1 in non-pregnant women; oestrogen in pregnancy changes this, with AVM relatively more common.

267 **T**

268 **F** – antenatal > puerperium > labour (2%) for berry aneurysms. Note that in obstetric patients most subarachnoid haemorrhage (SAH) is due to AVMs, not berry aneurysms. SAH mostly strikes in puerperium ×20 risk.

269 **T** – especially in the third trimester.

270 **T**

271 **F** – its use can be justified after the first trimester in some cases.

272 **T**

273 **T**

274 **T**

275 **F** – younger obese women.

276 **F** – tends to worsen.

277 **T**

278 **T** – thiazides can also be used.

279 **T**

280 **T**

281 **F** – rarely; the majority are unilateral.

282 **F** – anterior two-thirds – the chorda tympani.

283 **T** – the patient is unable to wrinkle their forehead – therefore, lower motor neuron.

284 **F** – it is associated with Tinel's sign – lightly percussing the nerve to elicit symptoms. (Cullen's sign is periumbilical bruising and oedema, which is associated with ectopic pregnancy.)

285 **T** – and also associated with rheumatoid arthritis.

286 **T**

287 **T**

288 **F**

289 **T**

290 **F** – smooth muscle is unaffected.

291 **T** – it is associated with congenital myotonic dystrophy.

292 **T**

293 **T**

294 **T**

295 **T**

296 **F** – avoid general anaesthetic if possible; regional is preferred.
297 **F** – there is increased relapse post-partum.
298 **T**
299 **T**
300 **T**
301 **T**
302 **T**
303 **T**
304 **T**
305 **T**
306 **T**
307 **F**
308 **F**
309 **F** – carboprost prostaglandin F2alpha can cause bronchospasm.
310 **F**
311 **F** – magnesium sulphate is used to treat severe asthma.
312 **T**
313 **T** – give pyridoxine when prescribing isoniazid.
314 **F** – 8th cranial nerve (not 7th) damage can result in deafness, therefore is not used in pregnancy.
315 **T**
316 **T** – maternal hypercalcaemia.
317 **F** – occurs 5–14 days after birth.
318 **T** – most cases of cystic fibrosis involve the pancreas.
319 **T**
320 **T** – there is a high prevalence of glucose intolerance among women with CF.
321 **T**
322 **T**
323 **T**
324 **T** – because of hyposplenism.
325 **T**
326 **T**
327 **T**
328 **T**
329 **F** – are still prone to crises.
330 **T** – unless there is iron deficiency anaemia.
331 **T**

332 **F** – hyposplenism is the rule. Only 5% will develop splenomegaly.

333 **T**

334 **T** – give 5 mg folic acid daily; there is increased red cell turnover.

335 **T** – resulting from blood transfusion.

336 **T** – chronic haemolysis.

337 **T** – secondary to infection. Parvovirus red cell aplasia.

338 **T**

339 **T**

340 **T** – precipitous fall in haemoglobin. Acute abdominal pain with rapid enlargement of spleen. Less than 5% develop splenomegaly as most have hyposplenism. Splenic sequestration more common in HbSC.

341 **T**

342 **T**

343 **T**

344 **F** – alpha-thalassaemia major.

345 **F** – beta-thalassaemia major sufferers are more likely to be of small stature and have a small pelvis and therefore require caesarean section.

346 **F** – avoid.

347 **T**

348 **T**

349 **T**

350 **T**

351 **F** – thrombocythaemia resulting from splenectomy.

352 **T**

353 **T** – seen in thrombotic thrombocytopenic purpura.

354 **T**

355 **T** – acute fatty liver of pregnancy is commonly associated with maternal obesity/primigravidae/multiple pregnancy.

356 **T**

357 **T**

358 **F** – changes seen are usually central with periportal sparing and very little necrosis; instead steatosis is predominant feature.

359 **T**

360 **T**

361 **T**

362 **F** – pulmonary hypertension.

363 **T**

364 **F** – mid-diastolic.

365 **T**

366 **T**

367 **F** – in the last month to 5 months post-partum.

368 **T**

369 **T**

370 **T**

371 **T**

372 **F** – 85%.

373 **F** – is not caused by vitamin deficiency but by osmotic effect of hyponatrae-mia and too-rapid correction.

374 **T** – resulting from central pontine myelinolysis.

375 **T** – vitamin B1 deficiency and untreated Wernicke's encephalopathy.

376 **F** – alkalosis.

377 **F** – 40% will develop UTI and 30% pyelonephritis.

378 **T**

379 **T** – hypovolaemia or sepsis leads to transient acute tubular necrosis; how-ever, in pregnant women, there is a greater risk of ACN (with serious permanent sequelae) and the risk of ACN is even greater if there is concomitant pre-eclampsia/HELLP (Haemolysis, Elevated Liver enzymes and Low Platelet count) syndrome.

380 **F**

381 **T**

382 **T** – women with retinopathy therefore increased risk.

383 **F** – tends to worsen with strict glycaemic control.

384 **T** – 33% per 1% drop in HbA_{1c}.

385 **T**

386 **T**

387 **T** – also increased risk of adverse pregnancy outcome if renal involvement/hypertension/lupus anticoagulant/anticardiolipin/first presentation of SLE in pregnancy.

388 **F** – anti-DNA rises and there is also a fall in C3 and C4.

389 **T**

390 **F** – erythema multiforme is associated with use of nifedipine.

391 **T**

392 **F** – the side effect of oxytocin is hyponatraemia.

393 **T**

394 **T**

395 **T**

396 **T** – case reports have been published.

397 **T**

398 **T**

399 **F**

400 **F**

401 **F**

402 **T**

403 **F** – bilateral notching on uterine artery.

404 **T**

405 **T** – rare, less than 1%.

406 **T**

407 **T**

408 **T**

409 **T**

410 **T**

411 **T**

412 **T** – and also anti-epileptic drugs.

413 **F** – dizygotic twins.

414 **F** – dizygotic twins.

415 **T** – IVF is associated with an increase in monozygotic twinning.

416 **T**

417 **T**

418 **F** – but rarely reported.

419 **F** – unidirectional arteriovenous are likely culprits.

420 **F** – donor twin.

421 **T**

422 **T** – does not include serious neonatal morbidity (4%).

423 **T** – no RCT, but many cite retrospective data showing improved survival.

424 **T**

425 **T** – such as, uterus cordiformis, but didelphys/bicornuate are too restrictive.

426 **T**

427 **T**

428 **T**

429 **T**

430 **T**

431 **T** – 1:1000 – 1:1500 deliveries.

432 **F** – mentovertical (13.5 cm).

433 **F** – submentobregmatic (9.5 cm).

434 **F** – occipitofrontal.

435 **T**

436 **F** – early neonatal deaths only included; that is, first 7 days.

437 **T** – and greater than 40 years.

438 **T** – and acquired.

439 **T**

440 **T**

441 **T**

442 **T**

443 **T**

444 **T** – theoretical greater risk of fetal drowning, as getting out of the pool in the active second stage could provoke fetal gasping.

445 **T**

446 **T**

447 **F** – 75 mg daily is considered safe antenatally.

448 **F** – up to 90%.

449 **T**

450 **T**

451 **T** – there is no robust data to demonstrate reduction in cerebral palsy or death.

452 **F** – approximately 15%–20%.

453 **F**

454 **T** – few deaths after 24 hours.

455 **F** – clinical diagnosis.

456 **T**

457 **T**

458 **T** – low uterine myoglobin.

459 **T**

460 **T**

461 **T**

462 **T**

463 **F** – accrete and moles increase risk because of loss of deciduas basalis, predisposing the passage of vasoactive mediators into the circulation. Praevia per se does not increase risk.

464 **T**

465 **F**

466 **T**

467 **T**

468 **F** – physiological jaundice occurs in the first few days of life and is associated with hepatic immaturity/absent gut flora impeding bile pigment removal/breastfeeding but does not persist for more than 7–10 days. Prolonged jaundice, which may not be apparent initially, is due to hypothyroidism/biliary atresia/galactosaemia.

469 **T** – anti-C, E, c, e, Kell, Duffy.

470 **T**

471 **T**

472 **T** – jaundice occurring within 24 hours is always pathological and results from blood group incompatibility, glucose-6-phosphate dehydrogenase deficiency and red cell anomalies such as spherocytosis.

473 **F** – 7 days.

474 **F** – 6 weeks.

475 **F**

476 **T** – due to risk of seizures.

477 **F**

478 **F** – 38 + 0 weeks.

479 **T**

480 **F** – 3 months prior.

481 **T**

482 **T**

483 **T**

484 **T**

485 **T**

486 **T**

487 **T**

488 **F** – from 15 weeks.

489 **T**

490 **T** – if amniocentesis is done before 14 weeks gestation.

491 **F** – 20 gauge.

492 **F**

493 **F** – more common in the third trimester.

494 **T**

495 **F** – transabdominal or transcervical approach.

496 **T**

497 **T** – when done between 8 and 9^{+3} weeks.

498 **T**

499 **T** – owing to a smaller uterus and thinner placenta.

500 **T**

501 **T**

502 **T**

503 **T** – Cochrane Review for 'Antenatal corticosteroids for accelerating fetal lung maturation for women at risk of preterm birth'.

504 **T** – Cochrane Review for 'Antenatal corticosteroids for accelerating fetal lung maturation for women at risk of preterm birth'.

505 **T** – Cochrane Review for 'Antenatal corticosteroids for accelerating fetal lung maturation for women at risk of preterm birth'.

506 **F** – 24 hours after and up to 7 days after administration of second dose.

507 **F** – not significant.

508 **T**

509 **T** – as found in MACS (Multiple courses of Antenatal CorticosteroidS for preterm birth) trial.

510 **F** – 38 + 6 weeks.

511 **T**

512 **F** – lower with betamethasone. Odds ratio 0.44 for betamethasone versus 0.73 for dexamethasone, $P < 0.05$.

513 **T**

514 **F**

515 **T**

516 **T**

517 **T**

518 **F**

519 **T**

520 **T**

521 **F** – less than 2 years.

522 **T**

523 **F** – male fetus is associated with unsuccessful VBAC.

524 **T**

525 **T**

526 **T**

527 **T**

528 **T** – according to the NICHD study.

529 **T** – according to the NICHD study.

530 **T** – 170/10 000 versus 100/10 000.

531 **T** – 289/10 000 versus 180/10 000.

532 **F** – no significant difference: 23/10 000 versus 30/10 000.

533 **F** – no significant difference: 4/10 000 versus 6/10 000.
534 **F** – 17/100 000 versus 44/100 000.
535 **T**
536 **T**
537 **T**
538 **T**
539 **T**
540 **T**
541 **F** – tachycardia.
542 **F** – no more than 7 days old.
543 **F**
544 **T**
545 **F** – not recommended.
546 **T**
547 **T**
548 **F** – blood loss of 1500 mL is anticipated.
549 **F** – this should be obtained.
550 **T**
551 **T**
552 **T**
553 **T**
554 **F** – 20%.
555 **F** – 3%–4%.
556 **F**
557 **T**
558 **F** – more than 3800 g.
559 **T**
560 **T**
561 **T**
562 **T**
563 **T**
564 **T**
565 **F**
566 **T**
567 **T**
568 **T**
569 **T**
570 **T**

571 T
572 F – no benefit.
573 T
574 T
575 T
576 F – microcephaly.
577 T
578 T
579 F – from 36 weeks.
580 F – from 37 weeks.
581 F
582 F – causes fetal bradycardia.
583 T
584 F – alteration in umbilical artery and MCA waveforms.
585 T
586 T
587 F – absolute contraindication.
588 T
589 T
590 T
591 T
592 T
593 T
594 T
595 T
596 F – late complication.
597 F – late complication.
598 F – late complication.
599 T
600 F – 5/10 000.
601 T
602 T
603 F – 6%.
604 T
605 T
606 T
607 F
608 T

609 **F** – fourth generation.

610 **T**

611 **T**

612 **T**

613 **T**

614 **T**

615 **F**

616 **F**

617 **F** – within 4 hours.

618 **T**

619 **T**

620 **T**

621 **T**

622 **T**

623 **T**

624 **T**

625 **T**

626 **T**

627 **T**

628 **T**

629 **T**

630 **T**

631 **T**

632 **T**

633 **T**

634 **T**

635 **F** – failure rate is less than 0.01%.

636 **T**

637 **F** – unreliable.

638 **F** – unreliable.

639 **T** – ~60%.

640 **T**

641 **T**

642 **T**

643 **T**

644 **T**

645 **T**

646 **T**

647 T

648 T

649 T

650 T

651 T

652 T

653 F – thrombocytopenia.

654 T

655 T

656 T

657 T

658 T

659 F – 0.1%.

660 T

661 T

662 T

663 T

664 T

665 T

666 T

667 T

668 F – should not be used in pregnancy.

669 T

670 T

671 T

672 T

673 T

674 T

675 T

676 T

677 F – 10%–15%.

678 T

679 F – 5%.

680 T

681 F – should be treated with laser ablation.

682 T

683 T

684 T

685 **F** – weekly.
686 **F** – at least 10 days.
687 **T**
688 **T**
689 **T**
690 **F** – evidence for this is inconclusive.
691 **T**
692 **T**
693 **T**
694 **F**
695 **F**
696 **F**
697 **F** – class III or IV.
698 **T**
699 **T**
700 **F** – 3 hours.
701 **F**
702 **F**
703 **F**
704 **T**
705 **F**
706 **T**
707 **T**
708 **F** – covering the internal os – not external os.
709 **T** – vasa praevia type 1.
710 **F** – associated with accessory lobes of placenta, vasa praevia type 2.
711 **T**
712 **T**
713 **T**
714 **T**
715 **T**
716 **T**
717 **T**
718 **T**
719 **T**
720 **T**
721 **T**
722 **F** – late age at first pregnancy.

723 **T**

724 **T**

725 **T**

726 **T**

727 **F** – until thirty-second week.

728 **T**

729 **F** – average number of movements is 31.

730 **T**

731 **F** – afternoon and evening are periods of peak activity.

732 **F** – no effect.

733 **F** – 70%.

734 **T** – 95% confidence interval 40–71.

735 **T** – relative risk 0·55, confidence interval 0.26–1.14.

736 **T** – relative risk 0.67, 99% confidence interval 0.45–0.89.

737 **T**

738 **T**

739 **T**

740 **T**

741 **T**

742 **T**

743 **F** – nulliparity.

744 **T** – up to 2%.

745 **F** – midline episiotomy.

746 **T**

747 **T**

748 **T**

749 **T**

750 **F**

751 **F** – until at least 12 hours.

752 **F** – until at least 24 hours.

753 **T**

754 **T**

755 **F** – could be given intravenously and subcutaneously.

756 **T**

757 **T**

758 **F** – 24 hours.

759 **F** – no activity has been found.

760 **F**

761 **F** – pentasaccharide.
762 **T**
763 **T**
764 **T**
765 **T**
766 **T**
767 **T**
768 **T**
769 **T**
770 **F** – slightly higher V/Q risk 1/280 000 versus CTPA less than 1/1 000 000.
771 **T**
772 **F** – routinely check platelet count when unfractionated heparin is given.
773 **F** – 2 years.
774 **T**
775 **F** – multiparous.
776 **T**
777 **T**
778 **T**
779 **T**
780 **T**
781 **F** – 7–8/1000.
782 **F** – 9/1000.
783 **F** – 4–16/10 000.
784 **T**
785 **T**
786 **T**
787 **T**
788 **T**
789 **F** – 5/100.
790 **T**
791 **T**
792 **T**
793 **F** – 11/100.
794 **T**
795 **T**
796 **F** – 26/100.
797 **T**
798 **T**

799 T

800 T

801 T

802 T

803 T

804 F – easier.

805 T

806 T

807 F – every 30 minutes.

808 F – every hour.

809 T

810 T

811 F – every 30 minutes.

812 F – every hour.

813 F – BP every hour but temperature every 4 hours.

814 T

815 T

816 T

817 T

818 T

819 T

820 T

821 T

822 F – benzodiazepines.

823 T

824 T

825 T

826 F – gestational diabetes and weight gain.

827 F – 1/2.

828 F – 1/6.

829 T

830 T

831 T

832 T

833 F – low.

834 F – low.

835 T

836 T

Answers
Gynaecology

1   T

2   T

3   T – hence salt-losing crisis.

4   T – accelerated bone maturation.

5   F – autosomal recessive.

6   T

7   T

8   F – majority.

9   T

10 T – 25% have short vaginal pouch.

11 T

12 F

13 T – 25% of cases.

14 T

15 T

16 T

17 T

18 T

19 T – but this is rare.

20 F – only treat if symptomatic.

21 F – if scarring present at posterior fourchette and/or new onset labial adhesions at 6 years or older may be indicative of sexual abuse.

22 T

23 T

24 T

25 F – malignant majority are unilateral.

26 F – second most common malignant ovarian tumour in this age group.

27 F – most common germ cell tumour.

28 F – 25%.

29 F – highest in post-menopausal women.

30 T

31 T – most often squamous.

32 T

33 T

34 F – less than 30 years.

35 T

36 T

37 T – most do not.

38 T

39 T

40 F – very often fatal.

41 F

42 F – less than 20 years.

43 F – these are dermoids with thyroid tissue and can cause clinical hyperthyroidism.

44 F – usually benign.

45 T

46 T

47 T

48 F – not known to metastasise.

49 T – eosinophilic bodies surrounded by granulosa cells.

50 F – precocious puberty.

51 F – can secrete androgens, but primarily secrete oestrogen.

52 T

53 F – only 5% occur before puberty.

54 T

55 T

56 T

57 F – 1%.

58 T – not all tumours produce these markers.

59 F – benign but usually occur in peri- and post-menopausal women.

60 T

61 T – Meig's syndrome.

62 F – older women.

63 F – does not secrete.

64 T – Meig's syndrome.

65 F – occur mostly in young women.

66 T

67 F – 80% 5-year survival.

68 F

69 T

70 T

71 F

72 T

73 T

74 F – 85% lifetime risk of breast cancer; 50% risk of ovarian cancer.

75 **F** – BRCA1 and 2 both confer lifetime risk of 85%; BRCA2 has 20% risk of ovarian cancer.

76 **T**

77 **T**

78 **T** – androgens are converted by adipose tissue to oestrone. Reduced SHBG.

79 **T**

80 **T**

81 **T**

82 **T**

83 **T**

84 **T**

85 **T**

86 **T**

87 **F** – 1% cases.

88 **T**

89 **T**

90 **T**

91 **T**

92 **T**

93 **T**

94 **F** – via blood to lung, bone, heart and liver.

95 **F** – less than 1% lymph node involvement.

96 **F** – variable; can be benign, borderline or malignant.

97 **F** – only from one nipple.

98 **T**

99 **T**

100 **T**

101 **T**

102 **T**

103 **F** – excellent prognosis.

104 **T**

105 **T**

106 **T**

107 **T**

108 **T**

109 **T**

110 **F** – clear cell adenocarcinoma of the vagina.

111 **F**

112 **F** – endocrine causes would cause secondary sexual characteristics.

113 **T** – *Shigella* vaginitis causes prepubertal bleeding.

114 **T** – tumour of the vagina can occur usually in those aged under 2 years.

115 **T** – tumour of vagina usually occurs in those aged less than 6 years.

116 **F** – not typically, as very rare to present without thelarche.

117 **T**

118 **T**

119 **T** – not rare in children and mostly presents as bleeding.

120 **T**

121 **T**

122 **T**

123 **T**

124 **T**

125 **T**

126 **F** – minimum of 6 hours.

127 **T**

128 **F**

129 **T**

130 **T**

131 **T**

132 **F** – less than 6/12 post-partum.

133 **F** – category 3.

134 **T** – cumulative risks.

135 **F** – category 3 if no other risk factors.

136 **F** – higher in nulliparous women.

137 **F** – absolutely UKMEC 4.

138 **T**

139 **F** – 20 mcg/24 hours. Contains 52 mg in total.

140 **F**

141 **T**

142 **F**

143 **F**

144 **T**

145 **T**

146 **F**

147 **F**

148 **T**

149 **F** – rifampicin is a potent liver enzyme-inducing drug. See Faculty of Sexual and Reproductive Healthcare Guidance (2011), 'Drug interactions with hormonal contraception').

150 **F** – 21 days.

151 **T**

152 **T**

153 **T**

154 **T**

155 **F** – not after 6 months post-partum in established breastfeeding.

156 **T**

157 **T**

158 **F**

159 **F** – every 8 weeks.

160 **T**

161 **T**

162 **T**

163 **F** – as barrier methods should continue for another 7 days after depot is given and another pregnancy test performed.

164 **F**

165 **T**

166 **T**

167 **F** – 3 kg.

168 **T**

169 **F** – no evidence of reduced fertility per se but delay in return of fertility.

170 **T**

171 **T**

172 **F** – primarily inhibits/delays ovulation.

173 **T**

174 **F** – no later than 120 hours.

175 **F** – may only be used once per cycle.

176 **T** – also do not use in severe asthma.

177 **T**

178 **T**

179 **T** – higher gastric pH decreases absorption.

180 **F** – progestogen in Yasmin®, which is a COCP.*

181 **T** – Cerazette®.

182 **F** – progestogen in COCPs Femodette® and Sunya®.*

183 **T** – Femulen®.*

*Progestogens used in POPs in the UK are desogestrel (Cerazette®), etynodiol diacetate (Femulen®), norethisterone (Micronor® and Noriday®) and levo-norgestrel (Norgeston®).

184　**T** – women with pre-existing migraine with aura may initiate use of a POP (UKMEC 2).

185　**T**

186　**T**

187　**F** – it takes 48 hours before the progestogen effect on cervical mucus has been restored. Remember that emergency contraception will be required if sexual intercourse has taken place in this 48-hour period.

188　**F** – UKMEC 2 but with lupus anticoagulant is UKMEC 4.

189　**F** – UKMEC 3; UKMEC 4 if 15 or more cigarettes per day.

190　**F** – occur prior to onset of headache.

191　**F**

192　**T**

193　**T**

194　**T**

195　**T**

196　**F** – in first week and UPSI occurred in week 1 or during the pill-free week.

197　**T**

198　**F** – can be, provided Fraser criteria are met: the patient understands the advice, will continue to have sex, is advised to inform parents and it is deemed in their best interest.

199　**T** – compared with an IUD which will prevent 99%. IUDs with banded copper on the arms with a surface area of at least 380 mm² have lowest failure rates.

200　**T** – all liver enzyme-inducing drugs may reduce efficacy, therefore a double dose is recommended. Inducers include: rifampicin, St John's wort, griseofulvin, carbamazepine, barbiturates, primidone, topiramate, oxcarbazepine and some antiretrovirals.

201　**T**

202　**F** – can use X-ray or ultrasound and proceed to HSG in selected patients or use HSG routinely.

203　**T**

204　**T**

205　**T**

206　**T**

207 **F** – complex quadraphasic regimen. Continuous 28-day cycle with 26 active and 2 placebo tablets with decreasing oestrogen and increasing progestogen doses.

208 **T**

209 **T**

210 **T**

211 **F**

212 **T** – the application device is also different.

213 **T**

214 **F** – 3 consecutive weeks; there is a patch-free fourth week.

215 **T**

216 **F**

217 **T**

218 **T**

219 **F** – the ring stays in situ for 3 weeks.

220 **T**

221 **T**

222 **T**

223 **T**

224 **T**

225 **T**

226 **T** – if risks of surgical intervention to remove IUD outweigh the risk of leaving it in place.

227 **T** – causes virilisation.*

228 **F** – only in the XY karyotype.*

229 **T***

230 **F***

*Ambiguous genitalia in 46 XY can occur in partial gonadal dysgenesis, partial androgen insensitivity syndrome, defects in testosterone biosynthesis and 5-alpha reductase deficiency. In 46 XX, it occurs in CAH, *in utero* exogenous androgens and in placental aromatase deficiency.

231 **T** – stimulation using synthetic adrenocorticotrophic hormone (ACTH) raises 17-OH progesterone in CAH.

232 **T**

233 **T**

234 **T** – can assess androgen receptors.

235 **T**

236 **F** – can be left until puberty. Lower risk (3%) of malignancy.

237 **T**

238 **T** – high chance of malignancy.

239 **F** – CAIS is X-linked.

240 **F** – converts testosterone to the potent androgen dihydrotestosterone.

241 **T**

242 **T**

243 **T**

244 **F** – four to five times more common in girls.

245 **T**

246 **T**

247 **T** – 80%.

248 **T**

249 **T** – 80%.

250 **F** – gonadotrophin dependent.

251 **T** – granulosa cell tumour.

252 **T**

253 **T**

254 **T**

255 **T**

256 **T**

257 **F**

258 **T** – decreasing circulating oestrogen.

259 **T**

260 **T**

261 **F** – 20% have recurrent or prolonged bleeding.

262 **T**

263 **F**

264 **F** – 14 years.*

265 **T***

266 **T***

267 **T***

268 **T***

269 **T***

270 **T***

*Swyer syndrome: 46 XY (some have mutation SRY gene)/gonadal dysgenesis/no testosterone or AMH produced/female genitalia/uterus and tubes present/tall stature/high risk of dysgerminoma. Kallman's syndrome: delayed puberty/hyposmia or anosmia/Kal-1 gene/X-linked.

271 **F** – only low doses are used as high doses may cause abnormal development
     of breasts.
272 **F** – hypogonadotrophic hypogonadism.
273 **T** – encephalitis.
274 **T**
275 **T**
276 **T** – iron deposits in the pituitary gland.
277 **T** – may affect the pituitary gland.
278 **F** – delayed puberty. In males, ambiguous genitalia.*
279 **F** – hypernatraemia.*
280 **F** – hypokalaemia.
281 **T***
282 **F** – primary amenorrhoea.*

*Deficiency in 17 alpha-hydroxylase is a rare condition characterised by reduced
or absent gonadal and adrenal sex hormones with increased synthesis of
mineralocorticoid precursors. It is usually diagnosed in adolescents who present
with delayed puberty.

283 **F** – causes decreased prolactin.
284 **T** – increases prolactin.
285 **T**
286 **T**
287 **T**
288 **T**
289 **T**
290 **T**
291 **T**
292 **F** – Addison's disease.
293 **T**
294 **T**
295 **F** – consider karyotyping but offer to all aged under 25 years.*
296 **F***
297 **F***

*Premature ovarian failure is associated with autoimmune disease.

298 **T**
299 **F** – less common among smokers.
300 **T**
301 **T**
302 **F**

303 F
304 F
305 T
306 T
307 T
308 T
309 T
310 T
311 T
312 T
313 T
314 T
315 T
316 T
317 T
318 F
319 F
320 T
321 T
322 F
323 T
324 T
325 F
326 F – lower education.
327 F
328 T
329 T
330 T – in 25% cases.
331 T
332 F – local excision.
333 F – excision.
334 F – only if recurrent and widespread. If widespread, 5-fluorouracil can be used. The risk of transformation to invasive cancer is 5%.
335 T
336 T
337 T
338 F – cause genital warts.
339 T

340 **F**

341 **F**

342 **F** – left.

343 **T**

344 **T**

345 **T**

346 **F** – normogonadotrophic.

347 **T**

348 **T**

349 **T**

350 **F** – 20%–25%.

351 **T**

352 **T**

353 **F** – younger.

354 **F** – lean women are more at risk.

355 **T**

356 **T**

357 **T**

358 **T**

359 **T**

360 **T**

361 **F** – 1%.

362 **F** – balanced reciprocal translocation is most common.

363 **T**

364 **T**

365 **F** – deficiency.

366 **T**

367 **T**

368 **T** – the risk rises in heavy smokers.

369 **F** – most common is ampullary then isthmic followed by fimbrial then interstitial.

370 **T**

371 **T**

372 **F** – prognosis worse if AB.

373 **T**

374 **T** – 46 XX is greater than 46 XY.

375 **T** – paternal origin.

376 **F**

377 **T** – 69 XXX, 69 XXY egg (23 X + {23 X + 23 X or Y}) fertilised by two haploid sperm (dispermy).

378 **T**

379 **T**

380 **T**

381 **F** – most do not.

382 **T**

383 **F**

384 **T**

385 **F** – large for dates.

386 **T**

387 **T**

388 **F** – hyperthyroidism.

389 **T**

390 **T**

391 **T**

392 **T**

393 **T**

394 **F** – FAI = total testosterone × 1000/SHBG. As active testosterone includes both free and albumin-bound testosterone, total testosterone needs to be measured. Testosterone is not active when bound to SHBG.

395 **T**

396 **F**

397 **T**

398 **T**

399 **F** – DHEA-sulphate.

400 **T**

401 **T**

402 **T**

403 **T**

404 **T**

405 **F** – unproven unless diabetic.

406 **T**

407 **T**

408 **F**

409 **T** – struma ovarii.

410 **T** – rare – can contain gastrointestinal tract epithelium.

411 **T** – true but very rare.

412 **T**

413 **T**

414 **T**

415 **F** – later menopause.

416 **T**

417 **T** – atrophy.*

418 **T***

419 **T***

420 **F** – short-term.*

421 **T***

*Menopausal symptoms include depression, mood changes, decreased libido, insomnia and hot flushes.

422 **T**

423 **F**

424 **F** – not consistently effective.

425 **T**

426 **F**

427 **T**

428 **T** – unknown after cessation of HRT.

429 **T**

430 **T**

431 **F** – increased.

432 **F***

433 **F** – is suggestive not diagnostic.*

434 **F** – pH > 4.5.*

*Amsel's criteria for diagnosis of bacterial vaginosis are: (i) thin watery discharge, (ii) clue cells greater than 20%, (iii) pH > 4.5, and (iv) 'fishy' odour.

435 **T**

436 **F** – in 2%–3% of cases.

437 **F** – anaerobic.

438 **T**

439 **T**

440 **T**

441 **T**

442 **F** – pH < 4.5.

443 **T**

444 **T**

445 **T**

446 **T** – genital warts.

447 **T**

448 **F** – syphilis causes painless chancre.

449 **F** – associated with 'bubo'. Granuloma inguinale (Donovanosis), caused by *Calymmatobacterium granulomatis*, is characteristically associated with Donovan bodies.

450 **F** – up to 90 days.

451 **T**

452 **F** – non-specific tests such as the VDRL and rapid plasma reagin may be used both for screening and as indices of response to treatment. They both measure reagin antibodies. False positives include: infections (e.g. varicella, mumps, measles, CMV, HIV, pneumococcus), autoimmune conditions (e.g. SLE, idiopathic thrombocytopenic purpura, rheumatoid arthritis, Hashimoto's thyroiditis, primary biliary cirrhosis), malignancy and intravenous drug use. If the screen is positive, then specific tests should be used.

453 **T**

454 **T** – treatment of both primary and secondary syphilis can result in acute febrile reaction, headache and myalgia within 24 hours of penicillin administration.

455 **T**

456 **F** – exotoxin TSST-1.

457 **T**

458 **T** – streptococcal toxic shock-like syndrome caused by *Streptococcus pyogenes* has been described as sequelae to surgical wound infection.

459 **T** – 95% sensitivity and specificity.

460 **T** – more than 50%.

461 **T**

462 **F** – diplococcus.

463 **T**

464 **T**

465 **T**

466 **T**

467 **T** – pulmonary or gastrointestinal tract. Mostly from lungs.

468 **T**

469 **F** – fallopian tubes.

470 **F** – antiHBs is a marker of vaccination.

471 **F** – hepatitis B virus DNA.

472 **T**

473 **T**

474 **T**

475 **F** – this is a recognised complication of anterior repair.

476 **F** – this practice is thought to increase risk of dyspareunia post-operatively.

477 **T** – excludes intussusception of rectum.

478 **T**

479 **T**

480 **T**

481 **T**

482 **T**

483 **F** – with or without urge incontinence.

484 **T**

485 **T**

486 **T**

487 **T**

488 **F** – used Rx frequency.

489 **F**

490 **T**

491 **T**

492 **T**

493 **T** – previously, less than 2 cm in size.

494 **T** – previously, all lesions confined to vulva greater than 2 cm.

495 **T** – previously, just stage III adjacent spread to lower urethra/vagina/anus.

496 **T**

497 **T**

498 **T**

499 **T**

500 **T**

501 **T**

502 **T** – there is no IC stage.

503 **T** – this is the new staging for uterine sarcoma.

504 **T**

505 **T**

506 **T**

507 **T**

508 **T**

509 **T**

510 T

511 T

512 T

513 T

514 T

515 T

516 T

517 T – the second injection will be given 1–2 months after the first injection and the third injection will be given about 6 months after the first. All three doses should be given within a 12-month period.

518 T – this age group is typically in Year 8 in schools in England. There is also a 3-year 'catch-up' programme in place, which started in September 2008, for girls aged 14–17 years.

519 T

520 T

521 F – the vaccine does not protect against all types of HPV and is therefore not guaranteed to prevent cervical cancer. This is why regular cervical screening continues to play an important role in detecting potentially cancerous cell changes in the cervix.

522 F – another licensed HPV vaccine, Gardasil®, protects against genital warts.

523 T – but it does not improve survival.

524 T

525 T

526 T

527 F – post-menopausal.

528 T

529 T

530 T

531 T

532 T

533 F – COCP reduces risk of ovarian cancer.

534 T

535 T

536 F – not routinely given but swabs should be taken to test for sexually transmitted diseases.

537 T

538 F – deep dyspareunia.

539 T

540 **T**

541 **T** – pain on defecation.

542 **F** – greater than 4 cm.

543 **F** – GnRH agonist.

544 **F** – 1/714.

545 **F** – higher incidence in the Asian population.

546 **F** – 1/50 000.

547 **T**

548 **T**

549 **F** – 1/80.

550 **T**

551 **T**

552 **F** – to reduce the risk of uterine perforation.

553 **F** – neither is preferred over the other.

554 **T**

555 **T**

556 **F** – risk is two times more.

557 **T**

558 **T**

559 **T**

560 **T**

561 **F** – 50%.

562 **F** – 23%.

563 **T**

564 **T**

565 **T**

566 **T**

567 **T**

568 **F** – haematocrit greater than 45%.

569 **F** – hypoproteinaemia, low albumin and pathological third space.

570 **T**

571 **T**

572 **T**

573 **F**

574 **F**

575 **F**

576 **T**

577 **F**

578 **F**

579 **F** – type 2 diabetes.

580 **T**

581 **T**

582 **F** – with rigid hysteroscope.

583 **F** – with rigid hysteroscope.

584 **F** – with rigid hysteroscope.

585 **F** – with rigid hysteroscope.

586 **F** – required for female clinicians as well.

587 **T**

588 **T**

589 **T**

590 **F** – 10%.

591 **F** – 17%.

592 **T**

593 **F** – 80%.

594 **F** – 16%.

595 **F** – 5%.

596 **T**

597 **T**

598 **T**

599 **F** – 2%.

600 **T**

601 **T**

602 **T**

603 **F** – this is a complication of sacrospinous fixation not sacrocolpopexy.

604 **F** – this is a complication of sacrospinous fixation not sacrocolpopexy.

605 **F**

606 **F**

607 **T**

608 **T**

609 **T**

610 **T**

611 **F** – 4/1000.

612 **F** – 23/1000.

613 **T**

614 **F** – 2/1000.

615 **T**

616 T

617 T

618 T

619 **F** – 8/100.

620 T

621 T

622 **F** – there is no evidence in the literature regarding impact on future fertility.

623 **F** – 1–2/1000.

624 T

625 **F** – 3/1000.

626 T

627 T

628 T

629 T

630 T

631 T

632 T

633 T

634 **T***

635 **T***

636 **T***

637 **T***

638 **T***

639 **T***

640 **T***

641 **T***

*The new WHO (*Manual for Semen Analysis*, 5th edn, 2010) guidelines have revised the previously accepted normal values.

642 T

643 T

644 T

645 T

646 **F**

647 **F**

648 T

649 T

650 **F** – both appear to be equally effective in terms of increased pregnancy and live birth rates per cycle started.

651 **F** – it is unlikely to result in a pregnancy.

652 **F**

653 **T**

654 **T**

655 **T**

656 **T**

657 **T**

658 **F** – less than 3 cm.

659 **F** – up to 10 weeks.

660 **T**

661 **T**

662 **T**

663 **T**

664 **F** – 1/20.

665 **F** – 1/1000.

666 **F** – 1/20.

667 **T**

668 **T**

669 **F** – 1/20.

670 **F** – 1/1000.

671 **F** – 1/20.

672 **F**

673 **T**

674 **T**

675 **F**

676 **F** – 4 weeks post-partum.

677 **T**

678 **T**

679 **F** – UAE.

Answers
Statistics

1 **T**

2 **T**

3 **T** – mathematical property of the true normal distribution.

4 **T**

5 **T**

6 **F** – ±3 SD = 99.73%; whereas, ±2 SD = 95% and ±1 SD = 68%.

7 **F** – to calculate the SD, the variance and N (the total number of scores) are required. Standard (z) scores are calculated using the SD to show how far above or below the group mean a given score is located.

8 **F** – histograms are usually used.

9 **F** – bar charts are usually used.

10 **F** – this is the mode.

11 **T**

12 **F** – there is a significant *negative* correlation; that is, as one variable increases the other decreases. Negative correlation is represented by a downward slope (Figure 1) on a scatter graph. The correlation coefficient ('r') is close to –1. In positive correlation, high scores in one variable are associated with high scores in the other. Positive correlation has an upward slope on a scatter graph and has a correlation coefficient closer to +1. 'No correlation' means there is no obvious direction on the scattergram. With no correlation, r, the correlation coefficient, is closer to 0.

13 **F** – there is a significant correlation but this does not prove causality.

14 **F** – it is parametric. Spearman is its non-parametric equivalent.

15 **F** – this test should not be used for nominal or ordinal data, only interval/ratio level data; the Spearman can be used on ordinal data.

16 **T**

17 **T**

18 **F** – Type II errors are reduced by increasing sample size.

19 **T**

20 **F** – Type II errors.

21 **T**

22 **T**

23 **T**

24 **F** – should be used on two unmatched groups.

25 **T** – data in named categories, for example, male/female.

26 **F** – is non-parametric.

27 **T**

28 **T** – if the hypothesis predicts that the results will go in one specific direction it is one-tailed.

29 **T**

30 **T** – the questionnaire results in ordinal data.

31 **F** – this is a parametric test and cannot be used as the data are ordinal.

32 **T** – a/(a + c).

33 **T** – d/(b + d).

34 **F** – as sensitivity increases, the number of persons with the disease who are missed by being incorrectly classified as false negative will be reduced.

35 **F** – as specificity increases the number of false positives will decrease.

36 **T**

37 **T**

Remember: positive predictive value = a/(a + b). Negative predictive value = d/(c + d).

Index

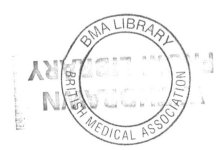